Terri Salt

REDUCING RISK
In Health and Social Care

TOWARDS
Outstanding
Teams and Services

Reducing Risk in Health and Social Care
Towards Outstanding Teams and Services

© Pavilion Publishing & Media Ltd

The author has asserted her rights in accordance with the Copyright, Designs and Patents Act (1988) to be identified as the author of this work.

Published by:

Pavilion Publishing and Media Ltd
Blue Sky Offices, 25 Cecil Pashley Way
Shoreham by Sea, West Sussex
BN43 5FF

Tel: 01273 434 943
Email: info@pavpub.com
Web: www.pavpub.com

Published 2023

A catalogue record for this book is available from the British Library.

ISBN: 978-1-80388-307-6

Pavilion Publishing and Media is a leading publisher of books, training materials and digital content in mental health, social care and allied fields. Pavilion and its imprints offer must-have knowledge and innovative learning solutions underpinned by sound research and professional values.

Author: Terri Salt
Cover design: Emma Dawe, Pavilion Publishing and Media Ltd
Page layout and typesetting: Emma Dawe, Pavilion Publishing and Media Ltd
Printing: Independent Publishers Group (IPG)

Contents

About the author

Terri Salt is amongst the most experienced regulators of health and social care in England. She has a substantive role with the Care Quality Commission as a Senior Specialist within the Commission's Regulatory Leadership team, advising and supporting operations staff nationally. She also has a part-time role as an independent chair of the final appeal panel for a local authority. Terri is a registered adult and sick children's nurse and coach, with postgraduate qualifications in public sector leadership, adult education, and healthcare. She writes for the *British Journal of Nursing*.

Terri is the author and Director of the *Towards Outstanding* brand, which is built upon the principle that all services can, and should, provide excellent care. It's about learning through reflection and sharing outstanding practice. The company is affiliated to Salt of The Earth Consulting Ltd, which provides executive coaching, keynotes, board development, organisational assessment and bespoke training packages for providers of health, social care, and education leadership. To discuss how *Towards Outstanding* could support your organisation, please contact terri@saltoftheeartconsulting.com.

Preface

"An ounce of prevention is better than a pound of cure."

Benjamin Franklin

As I began to write this book, I thought back to and remembered with pleasure some of the lightbulb moments that have helped me to understand safety and risk and where my personal risk threshold sits. Learning to manage risk and how to balance curiosity, independence and exploration with a desire to avoid harm is something we all face from birth. As a ten-month-old, our instinctive desire to climb steps because they are there is not balanced against any understanding of the risk of tumbling back down – that comes as we begin to explore more. Someone else probably assessed and managed the risk initially to keep us safe. Importantly, how that was done impacts on the child's learning of safety and risk. If a child is never allowed to climb stairs for fear they may fall, they may not learn to be good at managing their own risks.

Safety and risk management is a balancing act. It has to allow freedom to take risks for those with capacity to do so, but it must also have processes in place to protect against risks that the individual cannot reasonably be expected to consider or mitigate against. Fire safety in care homes comes into this category; it would not be reasonable for each resident to decide what fire-safety measures they wanted and needed to remain safe, so regulations were agreed that impose that responsibility on providers. A decision made by a very elderly person to continue to drive their car may be entirely reasonable, assuming their eyesight and reactions remain adequate. Family members may assume being aged means they cannot drive, but unless there is a genuine increased risk of harm to others, they should probably support the person to maintain their independence. Care home staff may face a similar need to address their prejudice if a resident wishes to drive and is able to do so safely. Safety and risk management are not about removing people's right to self-determination.

I have a moderately high risk propensity score. This is about my current tendency to take or avoid risks (which can change over time as a result of experience).[1] My score goes against the norm for younger people to take higher risks and for women to be more risk-averse than men. I put part of that down to a reasonably feral childhood where we took risks away from adult oversight. At four, I was going with my seven- and six-

---

1   Sitkin SB & Weingart LR (1995) Determinants of risky decision-making behavior: A test of the mediating role of risk perceptions and propensity. *Academy of management Journal* **38** (6) 1573-1592.

year-old sisters on a public bus to school, walking a mile at each end of the journey. We spent our spare time on the beach and followed the older children out to the raft chained in the bay, or onto the pier to jump or dive into the deeper water.

These are probably not things that most four-year-olds would be permitted to do now, but our mother worked in a beach café for the summer to put food on the table and childcare didn't really exist. I now take a small delight in watching seemingly confident teenagers hesitating before leaping off a bridge or sea wall into deep but calm water, then looking slightly horrified or amused at me hurling myself off. I learned at a young age to read the sea and the tides, to understand my limits and to know what I need to check before using a river, quarry, or unfamiliar beach to swim. There remains a degree of risk where deep or moving water is concerned but, for me, it's a measured risk that I have weighed up and am prepared to take.

As young adults, before we were married (and afterwards), my husband and I led holiday camps for disadvantaged children. We took up to sixty children away for a fortnight. We didn't know them when we met, didn't know many of the other helpers and there were no policies to guide us and no governance structure to monitor what we did. We were initially a touch blind to the level of risk we were exposing ourselves and the children to, perhaps. We learned pretty quickly, though, and I hope we offered a better, safer holiday each year we did it.

Lots of times stand out, but a key message I learned was about listening to people using the service. Yannus was a lad of about nine or ten. We knew his name quickly as he was a bit of a clown who liked being centre stage and making the others laugh. Lively. Lots of energy. Loud. A good footballer, too. Loved playing tricks and telling jokes. Especially at bedtime.

Yannus wouldn't settle one night. Shrieking and laughing at the same time, banging his head and shouting that he had a wasp in his ear. Jumping from bed to bed in the room shared with fifteen others. My husband looked and could see no evidence. Yannus was sure it had got in when he was swimming. That was about eight hours earlier. He hadn't complained at all since. Still he laughed, rolled around, and shouted he had a wasp in his ear. My husband asked me to look. I was a first-year student nurse, after all. Nothing to see, but he was keeping everyone awake and I did love looking at hospitals even then; I'd never been to Weston General before.

Off we went in the minibus, Yannus chattering away very happily. The doctor couldn't see anything either and reassured us that a wasp would have stung if it had got in the ear. We took Yannus back, gave him some paracetamol syrup and an ice-cream and told him to be quiet. He moaned all through breakfast but had become quieter and less engaged with others. Tired, perhaps, but also insistent there most definitely was a wasp in his ear. So we took him back to Weston General where a paediatrician was found. Then an ENT consultant, who said it was hard to see properly as Yannus would not sit still. He was admitted and his ear examined under anaesthetic. Next morning he was up, dressed bouncing around and wanting to return to camp. He was also holding a specimen jar with a very dead wasp in it.

Listening is so important to good outcomes.

Part 1:
Introduction

Disclaimer

I have written this book based on far too many years' experience of health and social care and regulation. Good care hasn't changed much over the years; it has evolved and become more accountable, but the underpinning foundations of compassion, kindness, teamworking, attention to detail and personal preferences remain as true today as ever. The regulatory framework has changes and is about to change again as the Single Assessment Framework is rolled out to all service types from the end of 2023.

This book is my work and has not been endorsed by the Care Quality Commission. I rather hope that there is nothing contained within that would be at odds with the views of others who work in health or social care or in regulation, and that the key messages allow reflection on how well a service meets the expectations of the legislative framework, but I am not going to tell you, in detail, how to run your service – and nor can I give you an unearned advantage in the inspection process.

Simply reading this book isn't going to get you an improved rating. I have no influence over that; there is a strict quality assurance and benchmarking process, whereby inspection ratings are agreed. I hope you do get improved ratings. If you are reading this book, the chances are we are on the same side and we both want people to experience high quality care.

The premise of the book is that providers and staff will reflect with honesty on how they deliver care and treatment, and then use those reflections to drive improvements. There are no guarantees: you and your staff must put the effort into understanding your own service, being honest about shortcomings and recognising the strengths you can build on. The book will hopefully guide you towards an understanding of where you need to travel, but it is not a free ticket. There is no easy ride to excellence. Indeed, putting the work in and seeing the fruits of your labours is part of the joy that comes with improved outcomes. It offers a way of thinking, not a replacement for thinking.

Information produced by public bodies in the UK, such as the Care Quality Commission, NHS England and the Department of Health and Social Care, is included and used in accordance with the Open Government Licence v3.0.

The licencing conditions can be found at:
http://www.nationalarchives.gov.uk/doc/open-government-licence/version/3/

Information produced by the Care Quality Commission can be found at:
https://cqc.org.uk/

All books and training materials in the *Towards Outstanding* series are intended to support services in England that are registered with the Care Quality Commission to provide regulated activities. They should have applicability to all sectors, and the material contained within them can be adapted to make it more relevant to specific organisations. It is not so closely aligned to inspection methodologies that it will become less useable as the way inspections are carried out changes – this will inevitably happen over time, but the basis of good care is timeless. The global impact of the pandemic has affected the way services are provided and regulated. There is likely to be a move towards more remote monitoring through the use of data and intelligence – which is why it is so important to have clear evidence of what you are doing well, and to share this through engagement with the regulator.

The book series does focus on the legislative framework for England, but with very little work can be adapted to be relevant in other countries which embrace health and social care regulation as a force for bringing about improvements, particularly where ratings are given. The Welsh regulations for providers of adult social care, for example, have significant overlap and include many of the same requirements as the regulations that providers of adult social care in England must adhere to. The Regulation and Inspection of Social Care (Wales) Act 2016 makes many similar requirements to the Health and Social Care Act 2008 (Regulated Activities) Regulations 2014. Scotland's Health and Social Care Standards are worded differently, but they impose very similar requirements on providers. The Regulation and Quality Improvement Authority (RQIA) operates in Northern Ireland and whilst its standards are, perhaps, more explicit, they set the same requirements. The framework for the Health Information and Quality Authority for Ireland has more in common with the English framework than is different. Whilst Canada has different guidance and standards for each province, the content is remarkably similar.

My experience and the case studies I include are predominantly from England. The messages are international and have relevance to most countries where health and social care is delivered with similar national or provincial standards. The list of English-speaking countries with aligned regulation frameworks is long and includes (in no particular order) Canada, Ireland, Scotland, Wales, Northern Ireland, Malta and Gozo, United Arab Emirates, Mauritius, South Africa, Singapore, Hong Kong, Jamaica, Australia and India. Many non-English speaking countries also have aligned regulation of health and social care settings too, particularly across Europe.

Good care is good care regardless of where it is provided. Excellence in health and social care has changed very little since I started training; it has always been about providing personalised care that meets the needs and preferences of individuals. The legal framework has changed, the level of accountability has changed, the way services are regulated has changed a little (but not as much as might be imagined) and the expectations of society have changed. Yet, if one reads the works of long ago, Florence Nightingale wrote: "The symptoms or the sufferings generally considered to be inevitable and incident to the disease are very often not symptoms of the disease at all, but of something quite different – of the want of fresh air, or of light, or of warmth, or of quiet, or of cleanliness, or of punctuality and care in the administration of diet, of each or of all of these." If slightly more modern words were used, the statement could easily have been written by any Director of Nursing in an acute or mental health Trust, or by any care home manager today.

From a medical perspective, Hippocrates himself said: "It's far more important to know what person the disease has than what disease the person has." The modern version of the Hippocratic oath says: "I will remember that I do not treat a fever chart, a cancerous growth, but a sick human being, whose illness may affect the person's family and economic stability. My responsibility includes these related problems, if I am to care adequately for the sick."

The basic underpinning tenets of outstanding care really have changed very little. We just need to remember them – and that can be challenging in our fast paced and ever-changing world.

Chapter 1: Beginnings

"I had come to discover that 'safe' was an illusion, a pretence that adults wrapped around their children – and sometimes themselves – to make the world seem comfortable. I had discovered that under that thin cover of let's-pretend, monsters and nightmares lay, and that not all of them came from places like the moonroads or the nightling cities. Some of the monsters were people we knew. People we thought we could trust."

Holly Lisle

I usually start a book, or chapter, with a quote. When I started looking for something suitable, I found pages of very apt words by the famous and the not-so-famous, an example of which is above. I think this is indicative not only of how important safety is in all health and social care settings, but also how complex it is. A further quote that I found reminded me of my training, a good few years ago, and how it linked to more recent work. The quote was "'Safety first' is 'safety always'", by Charles Melville Hays, who was the first president of the American Grand Trunk Railway.

I did my initial training at the Hospital for Sick Children, London. Our hospital motto was drilled into us each morning by our tutor as we sat drinking coffee and eating sausage sandwiches from a wonderful café around the corner from Great Ormond Street: 'The child first and always'. It was on the outside wall as you approached the hospital building, so not only did we hear it daily, but we also saw it. The message was repeated frequently, until it became part of us. We didn't think about it much at the time. We all wanted to stop babies fretting and make toddlers giggle by dancing to 'Agadoo' in the playrooms. We didn't want to have children crying themselves to sleep. We were chosen to train at the hospital because of that commitment and desire to see happy, well children and to provide support for their families during difficult times. The naïve view that nursing sick children was all about cuddles and pretty uniforms was quickly replaced with complex technical knowledge and an understanding that sometimes children are too sick to smile. What remained, though, was that embedded message – that everything we did, all our actions, should put the child first.

More recently, I have been involved in regulating Western Sussex Hospitals NHS Foundation Trust (now merged to form a completely different Trust) where the entire messaging around strategy, quality improvement, policies and practice was grounded in their Trust-wide philosophy of 'Patient First'. It was their True North. It was the reason they existed as an organisation, and that was very clearly understood by the staff across their hospitals. The focus of all decisions was on what was best for the patients.

The same is true with messaging about safety systems and processes. You cannot send a single email reminding staff that they need to lock dangerous substances away and expect that to happen routinely across a service. Safety messaging needs to be embedded, and that only happens if it is seen, heard and acted upon from the point of induction until the staff member leaves an organisation. During my training, the Chief Nurse and Chief Medical Officer saw the 'child first and always' message as they arrived to work each day, just as often as we student nurses did.

If you are looking for a book that provides a set of checklists and tools to complete, that tells you what tasks you need to complete each day or each week, then this probably isn't the right book for you. I aim to set you on the path towards excellence by sharing my experiences, what works in other services, best practice, a little research, and some things that form the Care Quality Commission published guidance. I will also highlight that, where there have been failings, there have also been consequences. Nobody wants to see people harmed because of safety failings, but it happens. Sometimes seemingly minor issues cause catastrophic events for people using services.

There probably isn't a doctor or nurse in the country who hasn't been asked numerous times what they would do if it were them, their partner, their parent or their child that the treatment or care options being described related to. Even as an inexperienced and very young student nurse, parents would ask us about their critically ill child. I think that is an important thought to hold on to and use. When thinking about what you would want from a service in terms of safety and the quality of care, what would you say to such a parent? Extrapolate that a bit and think about whether you would be content with the safety and quality of care in your service if it was being provided to you or someone you loved. That is the only benchmark that we as health and social care professionals should accept. It is certainly the key benchmark that providers should use and strive to deliver consistently.

In 2018, Healthwatch published a report based on their work with people using social care services.[2] Sixty-six percent of people who responded said that safety was of paramount importance to them. We often think that what is important is the softer stuff; the smiles, the gentle touches and the facilities. They are important, of course, but safety is the trump card. There is an argument that you cannot provide a caring service if you are willing to provide unsafe care and treatment. It is a choice for providers and registered managers. You may not be able to choose whether or not you have too many people in the emergency department to offer everyone a temporary space of their own in a curtained bay, but you can choose whether or not to escalate the matter and make changes to the service to improve the situation. You can choose whether or not to provide adequate

2   www.healthwatch.co.uk/report/2018-09-18/what-do-people-want-social-care (accessed August 2023).

staffing, equipment, screens and monitoring to ensure that the people lingering in corridors as they wait for a bed or a CT scan are as safe and as comfortable as possible, given the limitations you are working with. Excuses and blind eyes create avoidable risk.

A safety culture is about far more than a fire-safety logbook or fridge-temperature records. It is attitudes, values and perceptions that influence how something is actually done, rather than a list of rules or instructions on how it should be done. A policy remains just words on a sheet of paper or intranet page if it is not enacted by staff. And nobody will know whether the policy is enacted if it is not monitored. A poor safety culture leads to incidents (sometimes very serious incidents) and personal injuries (sometimes fatal or life-changing injuries). The organisational safety culture, the commitment of staff to delivering safe care and treatment and the effective leadership and governance of safety is probably more important than the purchase of safety systems, databases and equipment.

To demonstrate that your service, or part of a service, is deserving of an 'Outstanding' rating for the key assessment question 'is it safe?', you need to be able to show through robust governance that safe care and treatment is delivered every day – that the experience of the overwhelming majority is that they receive safe care and treatment. Excellence is not about innovative practice that sees a reduction in risk around a rare chemotherapy regime (although that is a good thing), it is not about a paramedic buying snow chains for 'their' ambulance during winter (which may be a good thing), nor is it about having a fully automatic defibrillator which features three programmed languages (also a potentially good thing). Exceptional safety is about the consistent and effective identification and mitigation of everyday risks for the service type. That might be falls reduction and pressure damage prevention in a care home or elderly care ward of a community hospital. It might be consistent completion of audits against the National Standards of Healthcare Cleanliness 2021 in an imaging department, or it might be good governance around food hygiene or medical gases.

Remember:

- Having policies is not proof of care delivery to the required safe standard.
- Having risk assessments is not proof of care delivery to the required safe standard.
- Mandatory staff training records are a good thing, but they are not sufficient evidence of care delivery to the required safe standard.

To be able to demonstrate that safe care and treatment is being provided, there needs to be the full circle of recorded and objective evidence at both organisational and individual levels.

A culture of reflection

I would venture that, if you are reading this book simply to learn how to get an 'Outstanding' rating without much effort, you have a long way to go. The best leaders are truly delighted to receive their rating, but that isn't their key driver. The only effective reasons for aiming towards an 'Outstanding' rating are to improve the care and treatment of the people using your service and to improve the working lives of your staff. It is, above all else, about being kind and wanting what is best for the people using your service, within your organisational structure and governance systems. Kind? Yes, offering a safe system is about being kind. It is unkind to ignore a frayed carpet knowing that an elderly person could trip and fracture their neck or femur. It is unkind to not wash your hands properly and pass norovirus on to an already unwell patient. It is unkind to dismiss a frequent caller to an Ambulance Trust call centre complaining of chest pain as 'same old story'.

Our own reflection should enable us to see and understand how well we and our service are performing in terms of safety. That honest reflection is vital to enable us to identify and mitigate against harms happening in the future. If we take a defensive stance, blind to areas of weakness, and start placing blame on other people's shoulders, then we will not see where we need to make changes to protect people.

Most leaders want to spread good news. To celebrate achievements and recognise innovation and exceptional practice. Saying 'well done' and building on individual and team strengths is both lovely to do and the best way to see those positive behaviours reinforced. There does, however, have to be a balance, and leaders and providers ignore at their peril bad news, staff concerns and reports that are not glowing. A leadership team who only wants to hear good news and an organisation in which staff who express concerns are dismissed as 'whingers' are likely to end up with a serious problem that they didn't see coming.

In 2015, the Kirkup investigation into the maternity unit in Furness General Hospital, Morecambe Bay, identified a culture of bullying and a failure by the board to face up to problems. One staff member who tried to raise concerns was referred straight to occupational health. The staff member reported that "It seemed that as I dared to raise a concern I must obviously be mentally unwell". The report found twenty instances of significant or major failures of care at the hospital, associated with three maternal deaths and the deaths of sixteen babies at or shortly after birth. The report stated that "The failure to present a complete picture of how the maternity unit was operating was a missed opportunity that delayed both recognition and resolution of the problems and put further women and babies at risk".[3]

---

3   *The Report of the Morecambe Bay Investigation* (2015) Kirkup B. London: The Stationery Office.

There are many examples from history where there has not been reflection, identification of learning points and subsequent changes made to reduce future risks. And as a result, tragedy has been revisited.

I suspect that few people will have heard of the Tek Sing. A beautiful ocean-going Chinese ship, the Tek Sing sank in 1822, in an area of the South China Sea, after colliding with a coral reef. As well as a large cargo of luxury goods, it was carrying 1,800 passengers. The following morning, an English East India Company ship encountered debris from the sunken vessel and an enormous number of survivors. The ship managed to rescue about 190 of the survivors and a small Chinese junk rescued a few more, but the rest of the crew and passengers remain in a watery grave. Over 1,600 people lost their lives due to the failure to sail a safe route because they were rushing and took a shortcut.

RMS Titanic sank in 1912. There is a well-established theory that a small coal fire was discovered in one of her bunkers (a not uncommon occurrence on steamships of the day). Stokers hosed down the smouldering coal and shovelled it aside to reach the base of the blaze, but it became uncontrollable after the ship left Southampton, forcing the crew to attempt a full-speed crossing. Moving at such a fast pace, they were unable to avoid the fatal collision with the iceberg.

Ninety years between two of the worst disasters at sea and the risk of rushing had not been learned. Yet tragically it didn't end there, and the real lessons were still not learned.

The Herald of Free Enterprise was a roll-on roll-off ferry operating between Dover and Zeebrugge. On an afternoon in March 1987, the ship set sail without the bow doors being closed and it became unstable as the water rushed in. Vehicles rolled from port to starboard and back. The ship capsized onto its port side on a sandbank, all its lights out, in just ninety seconds. There was not enough time to send an SOS signal, nor to lower the lifeboats or deploy life jackets and, consequently, 193 passengers and crew were killed. This incident did bring about numerous changes to improve safety at sea and also informed the Public Interest Disclosure Act (1998), which protects whistle-blowers.

Translating the risks of time pressures into health or social care settings, it is easy to see where pressure to get 'things done' and to work at an unreasonable speed, to cut corners to increase efficiency, can result in very poor outcomes and serious harm. Staff who have to get twenty-seven people to the dining room for lunch may not stop to check that a person's feet are safely on the foot plates of a wheelchair. Staff rushing to get people up in the morning may not clean glasses and check that hearing aids are in place, and so increase the risk of a fall. In fact, the whole idea of 'getting people up' is a risk in itself, isn't it? In Homes where there is a more relaxed, person-centred culture, where people choose what time to get up or choose to get dressed after breakfast, are likely to have better outcomes, and this includes fewer falls.

Ambulance staff rushing through vehicle checks at the start of a shift may not be very thorough, and may drive off to the first category-one call without knowing their defibrillator isn't working properly. Theatre staff under pressure to get through a complex orthopaedic list after the surgeon arrived a little late may take shortcuts around the WHO's Five Steps to Safer Surgery; the result may well be a 'Never Event' (an incident that should never happen if available preventative measures have been implemented).[4] If a provider gets a few 'Never Events' appearing on the electronic reporting database, then they are not only more likely to be sued or prosecuted, but they are also more likely to be inspected.

It is clear to those who have worked across several sectors that the highest-performing and safest organisations have much in common, regardless of the services they provide, their size or their complexity. Indeed, there are similarities with other organisations, which operate outside of the health and social care arena, where there is by necessity a focus on safety.

Cultures that inhibit openness and transparency tend to inhibit excellence, too. Listening to staff is important, whether you are a ward sister on a children's ward, an outpatients' manager, a care home manager, a practice manager, a superintendent radiographer or a paramedic.

This is probably a good point to reiterate that this book represents my own experience, knowledge and opinion and does not carry an endorsement from the Care Quality Commission (CQC), although I hope that few in the Commission would disagree with what I have written. I have led a range of services from children's homes to large teams of volunteers, from charities to wards and hospitals, from inspection teams to multi-agency resource centres. My thoughts and experiences about safety in regulated services have come from my own experiences and from the variation of safety and risk management in many different services.

This book is based on what I consider to be good practice. I believe the best way to improve is to focus on individual and team strengths, and to learn from best practice. We shouldn't ignore shortcomings – we should identify areas for improvement in ourselves and in our teams – but recognising and spreading 'good' works much better than berating people for perceived failings. Safety is everyone's business, and good risk management includes the views or concerns and involvement of people using the service, their friends and relatives, other visitors or professionals, the staff, and the leaders.

---

4   www.england.nhs.uk/publication/never-events/ (accessed August 2023).

The attitude and behaviours around safety and risk management of individuals impacts on care delivery and outcomes; it affects how people experience the service and has the potential to impact on their health and even their life. To achieve excellence, a safe culture must be disseminated across an organisation, gaining 'buy in' and ensuring staff (and visitors) are adhering to the agreed practices.

Really honest reflection about how things are done is an essential tool for driving improvements. Trying to demonstrate high performance by having a 'tick list' of evidence isn't the most effective way to ensure safety and build objective, measurable data that shows how safe the service is. I have lost count of the number of times that I have seen a hospital WHO surgical safety checklist audit or a care home handwashing audit that shows very high performance which is at odds with observed practice. An audit score of 100% compliance is a bit of a red flag that would lead me to sit and watch from a quiet corner. Audits are a very useful tool, essential to identifying gaps in good practice and improved compliance, but only if they are an accurate reflection of what is actually happening. Surgical safety checklist compliance is best checked by someone observing in theatre for a while. Handwashing can be observed as part of wider observations of care delivery; it is surprising to see 100% compliance results when handwashing sinks have 'very hot water' signs above them and no soap.

So, now to think about how I came to my understanding of safety and risk, and what the trigger is that makes me feel a service is 'Outstanding' for the 'safe' key question. It must be about the patients' or service users' experience and how standardised good care is taken to the next level to make it excellent care. That takes exceptional staff at all levels of an organisation. They must be educated about safety, supported to ensure they are able to deliver safe care, and given the resources to do so. It is not enough to have a brilliant executive team and mediocracy at other tiers of the organisation. It is not going to work if you have a safety-focused ward sister or care home team leader working against asset-stripping and chronic under-resourcing. Efficiency is good and can improve safety; inadequate funding and over-stretched resourcing cannot.

Excellence is about doing the basics well, every day. It is about systems and processes that underpin safety and risk management, and which can then allow innovation.

Part 2: Safety and regulation

Chapter 2: The costs of poor care

The journey towards achieving an 'Outstanding' rating is never ending – it is about understanding your service, reflecting on what you do well and building on that. It is also about recognising and promoting the strengths of others to build systems and processes that protect the people using the service, the staff delivering those services, and, of course, the organisation itself.

The staff? Yes, the staff. Very few people working in health or social care set out to cause serious harm to others. Yet harm happens. People die. People suffer life-changing injuries. Living with the knowledge that you have caused such harm, or at least contributed to it, cannot be nice, and many have resigned or given up their careers over such incidents. Some have gone to prison.

In the most recent published hearings, the Nursing and Midwifery Council have struck two nurses from the register. One had taken medication for personal use and the other had maintained a personal relationship with an ex-patient with mental health problems and then lied under oath about seeing them. Clearly, these two situations are both safety concerns, and in both cases the provider had acted to reduce the risk of harm to patients. Both nurses have lost their careers through foolish, unsafe behaviours.

Health care professionals may experience significant psychological effects including anger, guilt, inadequacy and depression, and may attempt or complete suicide due to real or perceived errors. The threat of impending legal action may exacerbate these feelings. Mistakes can also lead to a loss of clinical confidence. Clinicians may equate errors with failure, with a breach of public trust, and with harming patients despite their mandate to "first, do no harm".[5]

Sadly, five doctors died by suicide while under GMC investigation between 2018 and 2020.[6] That is five too many, and there is potential that appropriate safety measures by providers could reduce this risk and the tragic loss of life. An anonymous junior doctor wrote an article for *The Guardian* newspaper in January 2016, and I think it is worth quoting a section of her words:

---

5   Rodziewicz TL, Houseman B & Hipskind JE (2023) Medical Error Reduction and Prevention. In: StatPearls [Internet]. Treasure Island (FL): StatPearls Publishing. PMID: 29763131.

6   GMC (2021) Fitness to practise statistics and reports.

"On my morning drives to the hospital, the tears fell like rain. The prospect of the next fourteen hours – 8am to 10pm with not a second's respite from the nurses' bleeps, or the overwhelming needs of too many sick patients – was almost too much to bear. But on the late-night trips back home, I'd feel nothing at all. Deadbeat, punch-drunk, it was utter indifference that nearly killed me. Every night, on an empty dual-carriageway, I had to fight with myself to keep my hands on the steering wheel. The temptation to let go – of the wheel, the patients, my miserable life – was almost irresistible. Then I'd never have to haul myself through another unfeasible day at the hospital.

"By the time I neared the end of my first year as a doctor, I'd chosen the spot where I intended to kill myself. I'd bought everything I needed to do it. All my youthful enthusiasm for healing, big dreams of saving lives and of making a difference, had soured and I felt an astronomic emptiness. Made monumentally selfish by depression, I'd ceased even to care what my husband would think of me, or that my little boy would grow up without his mother."

Safety is about systems and processes – most of us have sat through cabin crew demonstrations of how to put a lifejacket on – but it is also about far more than that. It is about reducing risk by really thinking about the potential harm to individual staff and people using services.

The use of car seat restraints reduces the risk of a child dying in a road traffic accident. That is just a statistic, and in richer nations, it is still a fairly low risk. In the USA, for example, only 602 children aged thirteen and under died as occupants in motor vehicle crashes during 2014.[7] I say 'only' because there were 27,400,000 children under the age of twelve in the country in 2021.[8] My calculations work that out as about a 0.002 % risk of a specific child being killed in a car-related accident. Obviously, not all of those deaths were related to the lack of appropriate car restraints, so the risk of not fastening a child correctly is even lower. It would be possible to argue that the law around the use of safety seats and restraints was excessive for the degree of risk. Unless, of course, you were thinking about your own child, or grandchild, or a child you were caring for, if you consider that the statistics also show that 38 % of the children under twelve who died in a crash in 2013 were not buckled up. Over one-third of child deaths were possibly preventable by simply strapping them in. It's a 'no brainer', isn't it?

How is this relevant to regulated services that don't transport children in motor vehicles and don't fly their service users very frequently? Well, to take an example, in an acute hospital you might want to think about the World Health Organization's (WHO) Surgical Safety Checklist and how well this is

---

7   https://kidsittingsafe.com/car-seat-statistics-compilation/ (accessed August 2023).

8   www.statista.com/statistics/457786/number-of-children-in-the-us-by-age/ (accessed August 2023).

used in your hospital. I mean *really* used, as opposed to being an audit of records and a few ticks appearing as soon as it is known that an inspection team is around. Has everyone involved in perioperative care actually read the *WHO Guidelines for Safe Surgery 2009?*[9] It's a much more interesting read than the usual policy, and it puts into perspective why it is necessary and the difference it can make if carried out properly. Staff who fully understand why they do something are more likely to make it happen. Frequently repeating the message embeds it so that nobody would consider operating without using the checklist properly.

In 2008, a WHO-funded study in eight hospitals worldwide reported on the positive impact. Overall, following the introduction of the checklist, surgical complications within thirty days of surgery fell from 11% to 7%, and in-hospital deaths fell from 1.5% to 0.8%. Why would you not make sure it was followed correctly in your hospital or your operating theatre?

What about in care homes? They need personalised care, not institutional systems and processes, right? Wrong. Very wrong. They need to personalise care for individual residents, but providers and managers also need to have robust safety systems in place to ensure that they meet legislative requirements and, more importantly, that they keep people safe enough to enjoy that personalised care. Fire safety is a good area to think about, where a systematic and embedded check of fire-safety measures is carried out in the same way every time a designated person walks around the building. It's not enough to show that the extinguishers are in date and the emergency lighting works. Fire safety takes a bit more. It takes systematic oversight and an understood governance process. It takes a willingness to admit when things are wrong. Without full acknowledgement of a problem, there can be no resolution, and the risk remains.

At a very recent acute hospital inspection, I visited a ward because concerns had been raised about the security of the unit and the ease with which a detained patient could leave without challenge from staff. Entirely as a side issue, I noticed that the fire-safety doors were in a very poor state of repair with a significant gap between the two doors where an intumescent strip should have been. The provider, when told, denied an issue. They were asked for assurance and said there had been environmental checks. Knowing there were estate problems (i.e. problems with the building and premises) that were not being addressed to ensure patient safety, we informed the Fire and Rescue Service under our information-sharing protocol. They took enforcement action, and the issue was sorted – but how much simpler, cheaper and better for all involved if the provider had thanked us for telling them, reviewed all their fire-safety

9   WHO Patient Safety & World Health Organization (2009) *Implementation manual WHO surgical safety checklist 2009: safe surgery saves lives* [online]. World Health Organization. Available at: https://apps.who.int/iris/handle/10665/44186 (accessed August 2023).

doors and repaired those that were not fit for purpose? Luckily, nobody was harmed and there was a swift response to the fire service intervention. Sometimes it has more far-reaching consequences.

In May 2014, Morven Healthcare Ltd was prosecuted and fined £45,000 for multiple fire-safety failings. The home provided for seventeen residents including elderly people with dementia and disabilities. The failings included blocked fire exits, an out-of-date fire-risk assessment, an inadequate fire-detection system and the absence of an emergency plan in the event of fire. An embedded daily walk-around recorded by the shift leader or maintenance staff would have identified blocked fire exits or doors wedged open. There should also have been a weekly review of fire-safety evacuation plans, alarm checks and fire extinguishers in the correct place and in date. It might also have checked that fire-safety doors were in good repair and that evacuation equipment was in the correct place and also in good repair.

Morven Healthcare Ltd found safety failings to be expensive, but not addressing risks around fire safety can have far worse consequences. Fourteen elderly residents lost their lives in January 2004 in a fire at Rosepark Care Home in South Lanarkshire. A 2011 inquiry into the fire said that: "The management of fire safety at Rosepark was systematically and seriously defective. The deficiencies in the management of fire safety at Rosepark contributed to the deaths. Management did not have a proper appreciation of its role and responsibilities in relation to issues of fire safety." The inquiry report found that some or all of the deaths could have been prevented.

For providers of services, the risks are significant if they do not offer a safe service. In 2021, a care home provider was fined £80,000 after pleading guilty to shortfalls in catheter care and record keeping. In 2018, a care home provider was fined £120,000 following an incident in which a seventy-five-year-old woman was injured as a result of being trapped in a commode shower chair, resulting in significant injury which required surgery and left her with a stoma.

It's not just care homes that get prosecuted: Nottingham University Hospitals Trust was fined £800,000 after pleading guilty to two offences of failing to provide safe care and treatment to a mother and her baby, exposing them to a significant risk of avoidable harm in 2023.

In September 2020, the first prosecution of an NHS Trust was successfully brought by CQC. The prosecution related to the handling of the death of an elderly patient at University Hospitals Plymouth NHS Trust. The patient's oesophagus was perforated during an endoscopy procedure. The court heard that the Trust's incident report did not conclude that her death was a Serious Incident and so her family were not adequately informed about the death at that time. The Trust was fined £1,600 and ordered to pay legal costs of £10,845.43 and a victim surcharge of £160.

Services can be closed or suspended, and providers or managers can be referred to their professional bodies. This will have a professional and reputational impact, as well as a financial impact. I can recall many such cases from my own experience as an inspector, but two stand out. Both are genuine, but the first reads like it was a care home under the same ownership as the Fawlty Towers hotel.

Case 1: Mrs Green

Mrs Green had three care homes, providing care for about two hundred and fifty residents plus people staying for a 'holiday' (respite care). She disliked the term 'care home' and called the premises 'guest houses'. She felt that many of her guests were embarrassed that they had some degree of dependency and required assistance. We raised concerns, but they were dismissed as our lack of understanding about Mrs Green's wishes for a 'better class of person'. That was me told!

What our inspection found was not so much a can of worms as a container ship of worms.

- Mr Jones liked to breathe the sea air and take a daily constitutional. He sometimes became a little confused as everywhere was so busy along the seafront, but the police knew him well and staff always ensured he had a visiting card in his pocket so he could be brought back. Mrs Green told us that it was lucky the road outside was quiet and only one-way, so he could usually cross by himself. We met Mr Jones; he clearly had quite advanced cognitive impairment and was unable to show us where his room was. He didn't recall going out for a walk an hour previously, nor his ride home in a police car.

- Mrs White was a bit unsteady on her feet. She was provided with a golfing umbrella, as her walking frame was so ugly. Luckily, the home had very deep pile carpets, which, while making walking harder, cushioned the falls. Residents were discouraged from using the lifts; the staircase was a grand, sweeping affair which dominated the main entrance. Sadly, Mrs White fell when she awoke in the night, uncomfortable and confused. She had been in search of a staff member but there was only one member of staff in the building, and they were sleeping-in on call, rather than waking night staff. Mrs White suffered a subdural bleed and lost an eye as a result of the fall.

- Mrs Johnson was living in a basement room. She was very frail and too heavy for staff to lift into bed from her reclining chair. She was doubly incontinent and had severe pressure damage. She was allowed to remain at the guesthouse because Mrs Green was so kind and couldn't bear to see her end up in "one of those dreadful homes you hear about" (sic). Mrs Green understood that Mrs Johnson was embarrassed by her limitations and had ensured she had been left undisturbed by any contact from community medical or nursing staff. She had not moved from her reclining chair for over three months, with staff changing her bedding by tugging it out and pushing her from side to side to release the sheet and pads she was sitting on.

The thing the inspection team found most difficult to understand was how hard Mrs Green fought, running up very high legal costs as she fought closure. She remained completely convinced that we simply didn't understand.

Case 2: Dr Mirza

I was called on a Friday afternoon by the leader of an inspection team who was on-site at a cosmetic clinic. They had found serious problems and felt a bit out of their depth, so wanted support. I lived quite close to the clinic, so I grabbed my warrant and joined them. The clinic's USP was, 'The cheapest Butt-Lift in Europe'. We were inspecting because a London NHS Trust had notified us of a young woman developing sepsis and dying following attendance at the clinic.

The clinic was above a town centre convenience store. When I arrived, the lead inspector opened the door, as the surgical fellow who was with her was still in the operating theatre. I use the term 'operating theatre' very loosely. It was the front room of an unconverted Georgian flat. Stained, dingy blue carpet, window propped open with a door wedge. Filthy, fly-ridden windows and windowsills. Lying face down on a couch was a patient, wearing a blood- and serous fluid-soaked paper gown that covered nothing. They were conscious but feeling a bit nauseous. The untrained assistant went off to the kitchen to make her a cup of tea. I followed to ask about the service.

The kitchen sink was full of surgical instruments that the assistant put onto the draining board so she could fill the kettle. The surgeon, meanwhile, was on his phone sending emails. We stopped proceedings and transferred the patient to a local emergency department, where they were admitted and given intravenous antibiotics. The records had been falsified, the premises did not have planning permission, there were no records of drug procurement and a whole list of other breaches of regulations. The service was suspended immediately, and the provider was advised it might be best to cancel all future appointments. The clinic never reopened, and the surgeon was later de-registered by the General Medical Council and can no longer practice in the UK.

The point of these two examples is to show that, while regulation might be seen by some as overly bureaucratic, it mostly works to reduce risks where providers are acting in an unsafe way. It also shows that the risks of providing unsafe care are serious injury and death for people using services, and loss of business and loss of career for those who choose to provide unsafe care.

The financial costs of not-caring

If providers need more than a desire to ensure people are safe and reduce the impact of incidents, then there is also a financial incentive. Good, safe care really does cost less, regardless of the type of service. Between 1st April 2015 and 31st March 2020, NHS Resolution received eight hundred claims for incidents of retained foreign object post procedure. This cost the NHS £14,546,778.[10] I don't believe any of these objects was a wasp, mind!

---

10   NHS Resolution (2021) *Did you know? Retained foreign object post procedure* [online]. Available at: https://resolution.nhs.uk/wp-content/uploads/2021/03/Retained-foreign-object-post-procedure-Did-you-know-leaflet.pdf (accessed August 2023).

Figures supplied by NHS Resolution show that the NHS paid out more than £1.63 billion in damages to claimants in 2017/18.[11]

The costs of mistakes apply to all provider types:

■ In February 2000, the Court of Appeal awarded compensation of £362,377 plus costs against the London Ambulance Service NHS Trust when there were delays in responding to a person having an acute asthma attack.[12]

■ In 2019, a Scottish care home company was fined more than half a million pounds after one of its residents choked on a piece of doughnut and died. The resident had been assessed as being at high risk of choking and consequently was on a 'minced and moist/fork mashable' diet.[13]

■ In 2016, a GP practice was fined £40,000 by the Information Commissioner's Office for disclosing a woman's confidential details to her ex-husband.[14]

■ In 2021, an independent hospital was ordered to pay £20,000 after it delayed telling patients about a surgeon's bad practice, as required under the Duty of Candour.[15]

Of course, the financial costs are not just the result of prosecution. Caring for someone who has fallen, who has lost the confidence to walk independently and is in pain, who needs dressings changing or who cannot feed themselves with a broken arm, takes up far more staff time.

In services where poor care is accepted, there is a higher attrition rate for staff. Workplace culture has been offered as the fourth most common reason that staff leave the NHS, after retirement and relocation. Staff like to be able to provide good care; very few entered health and social care for the money or working hours. High attrition rates add to the risks and also add to the costs.

Money matters, of course, but more importantly – and central to good, safe care – is a culture that recognises and hears the voices of the people using services. Listening to them reminds me why I and many others working

---

11 MDDUS (2018) *NHS litigation costs continue to rise* [online]. Available at: www.mddus.com/resources/resource-library/news-digest/2018/july/nhs-litigation-costs-continue-to-rise#: ~ :text = NHS%20litigation%20costs%20continue%20to%20rise. %20THE%20 cost,2017%2F18%2C%20an%20increase%20from%20%20%C2%A31.08%20billion%20in%20 2016%2F17 (accessed August 2023).

12 [2001] QB 36; [2000] 2 WLR 1158; [2000] 2 All ER 474; [2000] PIQR P57; [2000] Lloyd's Rep Med 109; (2000) 97(7) LSG 41.

13 BBC News (2022) *Tullibody care home resident choked to death on doughnut* [online]. Available at: www.bbc.co.uk/news/uk-scotland-tayside-central-59973233 (accessed August 2023).

14 Bevan Brittan (2016) *GP Practice Fined £40,000 for data protection breach* [online]. Available at: www.bevanbrittan.com/insights/articles/2016/gp-practice-fined-40-000-for-data-protection-breach/ (accessed August 2023).

15 www.bbc.co.uk/news/uk-england-leeds-56931154 (accessed August 2023).

in regulation do the job we do. Why safety is so important. Why nobody should dismiss a poor culture and inadequate resourcing.

There are few more powerful words than those taken from the coroner in his concluding statement about the avoidable death of baby Harry Richford at East Kent Hospitals NHS Foundation Trust. He said:

"The poet John Donne wrote 'any man's death diminishes me' ... if that is true how much more are we all diminished by the death of a newborn baby. Today Harry should be almost two years and three months old. He should be a bundle of energy causing no end of mischief as a happy active young child. Instead his family are grieving and will no doubt for the rest of their lives. What makes it worse is that they are grieving for a child they do not believe should have died. I agree with them. Harry's death was in my judgement wholly avoidable. Mr and Mrs Richford were failed by the hospital, but more importantly Harry was failed."

Chapter 3: Changes to the regulation of care services

The regulation of health and social care services in England is changing, and a single assessment framework is being introduced. Some things will remain the same and the focus of work by the Care Quality Commission (CQC) continues to be about ensuring that people using services receive good care. The new regulatory platform is being rolled out, and the first changes that providers will notice are likely to be seen around autumn 2023, with more and more aspects of regulation being moved to the new system and new framework. Initially, it will be things like statutory notifications, where providers will not notice many changes but recording will be on the new system. Eventually, CRM, the current system for storing provider contact and records, will be turned off.

The five key questions remain:

■ Are services safe?
■ Are services effective?
■ Are services caring?
■ Are services responsive?
■ Are services well-led?

The ratings also remain, and services will continue to be required to display these on websites and within the service. The four levels of rating remain as 'Outstanding', 'Good', 'Requires Improvement' and 'Inadequate'.

What is changing is the introduction of new 'Quality Statements'. These are the overarching judgement about areas of practice. They are 'we' statements; commitments that providers, commissioners and system leaders should live up to, and which show what is needed to deliver high-quality, person-centred care. They will still be underpinned by key lines of enquiry (KLOEs) and prompts, but they will be the focus for reporting. The single assessment framework will be used in all types of services and will offer a consistent approach to judging the quality of care across all sectors. The new single assessment framework will consist of one explicit set of expectations, making it easier to establish a consistent understanding of what defines 'high-quality' care and a good service.

It would be fair to say that the single assessment framework remains a work in progress, and it has not yet been fully rolled out across all services. There have been some delays, as the complexities of using it for some service types are identified and the framework is tweaked to accommodate the wide range of provider types. Where it is not in use, the current inspection framework continues to be used. In truth, the specific framework used isn't really that important; high-quality care and treatment remains high-quality care and treatment regardless of the structure used by the regulator to assess that quality. Not supporting people to eat or drink enough has always been poor care, as has failing to respond to people's pain. That will never change, and if providers keep the people who use their service as the focus of what they do – if they talk to those people or their representatives and make changes when necessary – then the framework will fit around how they are working.

Local authorities and Integrated Care Systems will now be regulated, and they will be assessed against a subset of the Quality Statements.

The evidence collected and used to make judgements about the quality of service provided will be divided into six specific areas, in an effort to increase consistency, bring greater objectivity and deliver a more structured approach.

These six areas of evidence will be:

- people's experiences
- feedback from staff and leaders
- observations of care
- feedback from partners
- processes
- outcomes of care

While the framework will be standardised across all service types, the type of evidence collected and reported on will differ depending on the type of service and what is already known about them. Information required for registration may be different to that required for an assessment.

Evidence collected under feedback from staff and leaders is likely to be a direct discussion with staff and leaders who are working in a small travel vaccination clinic, whereas in a large mental health Trust it is likely to include the NHS staff survey and Workforce Race Equality Standards as well as local survey results. Staff discussions may take place in focus groups or by offering drop-in sessions.

Outcomes of care will be balanced against observed care in bigger services. Teams won't usually be observing or able to offer a critique of how well a caesarean section is performed, but they will continue to use the data around maternity outcomes and may choose to consider the number of elective versus emergency sections. Observed care will be represented proportionally. Two people observed to be in wet and soiled clothes in a care home may be more significant than two people in wet and soiled clothes in a very large emergency department. The observations will be reflective of the situation. Nobody should be left in wet or soiled clothes, but the people in the emergency department may have just arrived with their clothes in that state or may have refused to allow staff to help them change. In a GP practice, outcome data is likely to be more significant than in a small travel clinic.

Currently, the Commission carries out an assessment of a service by way of an inspection. This is the only way ratings may be changed and a report of quality published. The inspection leads to judgements in the five key questions and then an overall rating is given. While inspections will remain an important part of CQC assessment, the new regulatory model offers a rolling assessment of quality and risk. This means that inspections will not be the only way that CQC assess a service. They will become a part of a broader style of ongoing assessment that will include:

- different ways of understanding the experiences of people using services.
- information from staff and leaders.
- direct monitoring activities – usually a structured phone conversation and evidence request.
- evidence providers submit via the CQC portal.
- surveys and focus groups.

Each area of an assessment can result in a rating change. CQC intend to assess and update their information about all aspects of services at least every two years.

Site visits (inspections) will still take place. CQC want to form a picture of how well a service is being provided over time, offering a more up-to-date view of quality and safety. This should result in a greater ability to identify and respond to emerging risk

The operational teams at the Commission are also changing, and in preparation for a greater focus on how systems deliver care and complex care pathways, the staff are moving into teams that have inspectors from each sector working together. These new teams will be made up of assessors, inspectors, regulatory co-ordinators and regulatory officers. An operations manager will lead each team. Depending on the services in a particular area, teams will contain a mix of the following roles:

- Assessors: whose role is to ensure that the Commission has an ongoing view of quality, safety and risk for services in their area. Supported by the inspector and regulatory co-ordinator, they will make judgements about the quality of care. To do this, they will consider evidence collected from all sources – both on and off-site.

- Inspectors: to lead any enforcement activity. While assessors will collect evidence off-site, inspectors will gather evidence during site visits (inspections).

- Regulatory co-ordinators: to help carry out engagement with providers and local groups of people. They will help with triaging information and collecting evidence.

- Regulatory officers: to support administrative duties. For example, inspection planning and gathering the experiences of people using services.

A regulatory leadership team has also been created, with senior specialists offering advice and support to operational teams on more complex issues. As well as primary medical services, adult social care and secondary and specialist care, there will be sub-teams for safeguarding and closed cultures, children's services, and integrated care.

For providers, this means:

- They will still be assessed by staff who understand the service they are assessing and inspecting.

- The traditional model of the relationship owner engaging with the provider will loosen. Providers and managers will be able to speak with different members of local teams for different types of advice, and rely less on one person to provide support. This might mean that a person with good knowledge about the Mental Health Act requirements is best placed to speak to an acute hospital about a detained person, but a care home manager speaks to someone with oversight of an acute Trust about poor discharge arrangements. The finer details or who will build the essential relationships with NHS Trusts and other very large providers has yet to be finalised.

There is an intention for the Commission to have an up-to-date view of quality and a better understanding of what is driving poor or excellent care in a particular area. Things like ambulance delays or emergency department delays can be understood better when they are considered as part of a system-wide provision. Poor health outcomes are better understood when the entire journey is considered; care and treatment often follow a pathway through multiple providers, with each having responsibility and an impact on the overall quality of care.

Risk-based inspections and ratings changes

The rating system will remain, but it is likely to be more fluid as policy changes result in the Commission changing ratings without a comprehensive inspection taking place. Until now, focused inspections and reviews did not usually result in a ratings change. Moving forward, a focused inspection of a part of a service, of one of the provider's locations or around a specific area of practice, may mean changes to the provider ratings. Those changes will not only be about the area of the service inspected or reviewed; they may also be aggregated into the overall location or provider rating.

A recent example is the maternity review programme – a national review carried out by a specialist team. In 2016, the then-Chief Inspector of Hospitals, Professor Sir Mike Richards, responded to the National Maternity Review: "As the report makes clear, every single woman deserves to receive personalised care that is based around their individual needs and decisions when having a baby. This is echoed in the findings from CQC's latest national maternity survey, which reinforce the importance of NHS Trusts focusing on women's individual needs and choices."

Since then, several high-profile cases have led to inquiries by experts appointed by the government. This includes the report of the independent investigation led by Dr Bill Kirkup, *Maternity and neonatal services in East Kent: 'Reading the signals' report*.[16] The report set out the truth of what happened so that maternity services in East Kent could begin to meet the standards expected nationally and prevent further harm, and it identified four areas for action. Earlier in 2022, the Ockenden Report was published.[17] The investigation, chaired by Donna Ockenden, was a government-commissioned Independent Maternity Review of maternity services at the Shrewsbury and Telford Hospital NHS Trust. The Trust failed to investigate, failed to learn and failed to improve, and therefore often failed to safeguard mothers and their babies at one of the most important times in their lives.

The Care Quality Commission responded to the concerns raised in both reports and set up a specialist team to review how Trusts had responded to the recommendations in the Ockenden Report and to gather an accurate and current picture of how maternity services were being delivered across the country. The review is ongoing at the time of writing, but it has identified a number of maternity services where there are significant safety and leadership concerns. Some of these services were rated as 'Good' from their

16 https://www.gov.uk/government/publications/maternity-and-neonatal-services-in-east-kent-reading-the-signals-report accessed 24/3/2023 www.gov.uk/government/publications/maternity-and-neonatal-services-in-east-kent-reading-the-signals-report (accessed August 2023).

17 www.gov.uk/government/publications/final-report-of-the-ockenden-review/ockenden-review-summary-of-findings-conclusions-and-essential-actions (accessed August 2023).

most recent comprehensive inspection. The maternity services ratings were aggregated into the overall hospital and Trust ratings and, in many cases, supported a 'Good' rating overall.

Where the maternity review team found concerns and identified care failings, a Rating Agreement Meeting was held, chaired by a director. In several cases, the Trust found their previous 'Good' rating was downgraded to 'Requires Improvement' or even 'Inadequate' for the 'safe' domain. The way the aggregation tool works is that this feeds first into the overall maternity service rating. An 'Inadequate' rating for safety is limiting; the overall service rating cannot remain as 'Good' if the safe domain is judged to be 'Inadequate'. This lowered score affects the location rating and possibly the Trust's overall rating (dependent on the balance of other ratings), so Trusts have found themselves with a lower overall rating without a comprehensive inspection.

Similarly, it might be unreasonable to have a 'Good' rating showing for a care home where there had been a trend of deep pressure wounds over a six-month period, or where the local community nursing service raised concerns about a dirty home and several people had been harmed by a Campylobacter infection. If a focused inspection found that the home's infection prevention and control measures, including food hygiene, were not meeting required standards, then the rating might well be lowered until improvements were made.

People using services and their families and friends want to know that the rating the Commission publishes on their website is an accurate reflection of the service, to enable them to make informed choices. Waiting for the next comprehensive inspection before changes to the ratings can happen means that people are not always provided with current information about quality and safety.

The new ways of working at the Commission, the new roles and multi-disciplinary teams, mean that the information about a service will be monitored and assessed by different people. They will be looking at risk levels based around data and key information that is received from national audits and surveys, staff, members of the public sharing information, other regulators and professional bodies, and through the Integrated Care Systems. The increased focus on risk means that the higher the level of assessed risk, the more likely an inspection. If an inspection is risk-based, it is more likely to result in a lowered rating and possibly enforcement action. That feels like another good reason to keep risk levels low and ensure there is objective evidence that the service is providing safe care and treatment.

So, what sort of risks are considered?

There are the obvious harm-related risk indicators – a series of 'Never Events' on a critical care unit, an increase in high-level pressure damage or falls in a care home, an increased number of deaths in an independent hospital or an increased number of contacts by whistle-blowers. For most of these risks, the provider should both be very aware of the increased risk and taking action to reduce it and improve outcomes well before an inspection team arrives. Sometimes, the action taken and evidence of the effectiveness of what has been done will be sufficient assurance; the level of assurance and likelihood of inspection will, in part, be dependent on a robust response when increased risk or increased harm is identified.

There are also other risks that will be considered. Having a registered manager in day-to-day control of the service reduces risk levels and has been shown to lead to improved compliance. Conversely, not having a registered manager is seen to increase the risk of non-compliance. Longstanding and repeated non-compliance or outstanding requirement notices increase the risk scores. Of particular concern are services that 'yo-yo' into and out of compliance.

Some service types are considered to be higher risk because of the vulnerabilities of the people using them (such as services for people with learning disabilities and autism). Some are higher risk because the service type is statistically more likely to be subject to enforcement action or have lower ratings. Hospices are the service type most likely to have consistently high ratings over time and across the country; this lowers the risk level for a hospice provider.

Increasingly, the risk-level determinators will be data driven. This means the scores and the likelihood of inspection will be more objective. Higher-risk services are still likely to see regular (at least annual) visits, not necessarily because of any specific increased risk but because of the vulnerabilities of the people using them. In larger services and acute healthcare settings, there is greater scope for assurance from recent data, so there is, perhaps, a higher threshold for site visits.

Statutory Notifications

The Care Quality Commission (Registration) Regulations 2009 require that the details of some incidents, events and changes to a service, or the people using the service, must be notified to the Commission.[18] There is comprehensive guidance on the CQC website for providers. It is added in here as there is a link between incident reporting and investigation and statutory notifications, and there should be consideration of whether a

18   CQC (2015) *Guidance on statutory notifications ASC IH PDC PA Reg Persons* [online]. Available at: www.cqc.org.uk/sites/default/files/20161101_100501_v7_guidance_on_statutory_notifications_ASC_IH_PDC_PA_Reg_Persons.pdf (accessed August 2023).

statutory notification also requires to be reported through the incident-reporting process and vice versa. They won't always, but sometimes will, which is why it should be considered each time an incident is recorded, or a statutory notification is submitted.

For example, there is a requirement that the death of a person who uses the service (Regulation 16) results in a Statutory Notification being submitted without delay. The vague 'without delay' is the timescale requirement for a number of notifications. It means exactly what it says – that providers should submit their notification as quickly as possible after the event has happened. It might be reasonable and 'without delay' for the manager of a care home for people living with dementia to submit the notification of a resident's expected death when they are back from their three days' leave. It might be less reasonable for a private dentist to take that long if someone died following an anaphylactic reaction to a local anaesthetic. In terms of notifications about deaths, they are assessed as either significant or routine.

Sometimes, ticking a box incorrectly (e.g., 'unexpected' versus 'expected') can generate an amount of traffic backwards and forwards between providers and the Commission. Sometimes there is insufficient detail for a death to automatically be considered routine, and that can result in more traffic. It is best to put in the details and provide assurance about the circumstances. A large hospice provider may have a number of deaths in a week, and they might submit a block of notifications together that are all likely to be classed as routine as most people using hospice services are terminally ill. A notification from a care home of an elderly person with end-stage dementia dying surrounded by their family is likely to be routine. Conversely, someone dying following a fall with a potential link to a serious medication error, or a younger adult with learning difficulties being run over, is going to be significant and more information will be required. It isn't necessarily the case that this will reflect badly on the service, but such incidents raise questions, and enforcement or even prosecution for individual care lapses may be considered.

Most services need to notify the Commission of the death of a person who uses the service, regardless of whether it was a peaceful, expected death, an unexpected but not particularly concerning death (perhaps a person with a serious medical condition that had not been identified previously), an accidental death or one involving violence. NHS services do not need to notify deaths that are expected nor other deaths via the statutory notification process; they use the NHS reporting systems. The provider needs to determine what 'a person using the service' means in practice. It is obvious that a person living in a care home is 'a person using the service', as is a patient attending an outpatient appointment or having surgery in a private hospital. It becomes a bit harder when considering community-based services. Does a woman who is a patient using a private fertility clinic, but who tragically dies in a road traffic accident between appointments, count as 'a person using services'? Probably not. Does a person who is discharged from a mental health crisis team and who later completes suicide count as 'a person using the service'? Undoubtedly.

Each service is different, and each will need to determine within their Incident Policy or Reporting Policy what constitutes a 'person using the service'. Erring on the side of caution will usually be the best option.

Notification of the death (or unauthorised absences) of a person who has been detained or liable to be detained under the Mental Health Act 1983 must be submitted slightly differently. They are still on the webform, but there is a need for more detail as the Commission handles these notifications separately from other notifications because of its statutory Mental Health Act monitoring duties.

These statutory notifications are the legal responsibility of the registered manager, or provider: they will be committing an offence if they don't submit the notifications, whenever required and in a timely way. The task can be delegated, but the legal responsibility cannot – so the way the task is delegated and the person(s) responsible must be very clear. It is a good idea to have the details of what needs to be notified within the incident policy, so that it is not overlooked.

The notifications are submitted via an webform rather than in a paper format and are quite simple to use. The provider or staff member completing them needs to be mindful that they do not put in personal details that allow for identification of the individuals affected and consequently contravene the Data Protection Act 1998. Providers can allocate a code to each person to use in submitting notifications. This might, for example, be something like: "Service user SU2 entered another services user's room (SU5) and tried to get into bed with them until staff member RN1 heard SU5 calling out and persuaded SU2 out of the room and into the communal lounge". What code you use doesn't matter. Codes and what they mean (the people's details) should be stored securely in case the Commission needs them at some point in the future. Codes shouldn't be obvious – so using a person's initials and date of birth, for instance, wouldn't be appropriate. The best place to store a code is in each person's individual record. Maybe a dated entry, an incident reference number, and their code.

Most NHS services don't use statutory notifications. They use national reporting systems instead. There are exceptions – if the NHS Trust or provider has an adult social care service or an independent hospital on their site that they own as a separate legal entity, for example, or if a GP practice also offers an entirely private service outside of their NHS contract.

You do need to submit notifications if you are a registered provider or a registered manager of:

- independent healthcare service (clinic, hospital, diagnostic centre, consulting service)
- adult social care
- primary dental care
- private ambulance services (even if they only contract to NHS services and use their reporting framework)

There is no requirement to notify the CQC about all medicines errors, but a notification would be required if the cause or effect of a medicine error resulted in death or injury, was possibly a sign of abuse, or if the police were involved. If medicine errors are possibly a part of the cause (or effect) of a notifiable situation, then this should be mentioned on the form.

There is a requirement to notify the Commission about any change to the service's statement of purpose. This is not usually part of the 'safe' key question, but it can be. If an incident is investigated and the provider decides to make significant changes, such as stopping the treatment of children or perhaps closing a service as they do not believe they have sufficient staff to provide that service safely, then the notification is positive evidence of responding to an identified risk. It is in the provider's interest to make sure they are compliant and have submitted the notification. Any amendments to a statement of purpose must be submitted within 28 days of the changes.

There is also a requirement to notify the Commission about other incidents. Again, this must be done without delay, and you cannot wait to check with the registered manager when they are back from three weeks' leave. There should be details of who has delegated responsibility included in the incident or reporting policy. The requirement is for notification if the 'other incident' takes place while a regulated activity is being delivered, or as a consequence of that regulated activity. The incidents that this applies to are:

- **Serious injuries.** The CQC webform gives details of the injuries that are reportable via a statutory notification. This is not a sibling falling over at a children's hospice and getting a graze, or a person with a learning disability burning their finger while cooking.
- **Deprivation of liberty applications and their outcomes.** This is a requirement to notify of application rather than approval. The approval must also be notified, and the two can be done at the same time if the outcome is known in a timely way.
- **Abuse and allegations of abuse.** You must notify the Commission about abuse or alleged abuse involving a person or people using your service.

This includes where the person is the victim, the abuser or both. It does not mean where a practitioner becomes aware of abuse that has been identified and managed appropriately elsewhere – for example, a termination of pregnancy service that learns about historic child abuse from a woman using a service as part of their medical history does not need to complete a notification. The same service being told about female genital mutilation does need to notify CQC (as well as ensuring that provider and local safeguarding processes are followed properly). Notifying CQC is not the same as making a safeguarding referral. Any care provider who identifies abuse or potential abuse has an obligation to ensure that the correct referral processes are followed, and that the referral has been received. If there is any suggestion or suspicion that a crime has been committed then the provider, or its staff, has a duty to inform the police.

■ **Incidents reported to, or investigated by, the police.** If a provider is made aware, for example, that a member of their staff has been arrested for theft from elderly neighbours, then there is a clear risk to elderly people using the domiciliary care agency where the person works. That needs reporting to CQC. Hearing from a member of staff about a speed-awareness course doesn't usually – unless driving is an integral part of their role. Anything involving the misuse of drugs needs reporting, as does any act of violence. A family member arriving drunk, making racist comments, and causing criminal damage needs reporting – it also needs reporting after the police have been informed.

■ **Events that stop, or may stop, the registered person from running the service safely and properly.** The provider and registered manager need to be clear about what this means for their service. The scale and scope of the services provided will help inform the decision. If I think back to incidents I have seen under this heading, they include (but are not limited to):

   ■ a care home at risk of running out of food and heating oil due to financial difficulties

   ■ a private hospital flooding

   ■ a community healthcare provider reporting that snow was preventing staff getting to work and making community visits

   ■ a fire in a care home

   ■ an outbreak of norovirus affecting staff and residents

   ■ criminal damage to a provider's private ambulance fleet

   ■ computer gremlins

There are too many things that could be covered. Many can be mitigated by good leaders taking swift action to reduce the risks. Others require Integrated Care System leaders to become involved and offer practical support. In the case of the snow-bound staff, the community services provider was able to call in local volunteers with four-wheel drive vehicles, to work with other healthcare providers locally, to enable staff to work wherever they could get to (usually closer to home) and so swap roles during the worst of the weather. This saw practice nurses going out to dress wounds in people's homes and make sure elderly patients were warm and fed, community nurses supporting GP practices, and midwives being driven around in military vehicles. Collaborative working at its very best.

■ **The admission of a child or young person under eighteen to an adult psychiatric ward or unit.** Providers who run psychiatric units for adults must notify CQC if they admit a child or young person aged under eighteen, if that placement has lasted for a continuous period longer than forty-eight hours.

These are the statutory notifications, and they are a legal responsibility. Good providers who want to build positive relationships and be proactive in ensuring an accurate picture of their services will often choose to notify beyond this. Incidents that don't require a statutory notification can still be shared with the Commission through a call to the contact centre, an email, or by contacting the person that holds the relationship (if known). A 'heads up' along with details of how a situation has been managed and the risk reduced can save a greater regulatory burden later on.

Chapter 4: Know your service!

The first step in the process of ensuring that people receive safe and high-quality care is to know your service. That may seem very obvious, but it is often overlooked by providers, registered managers and leaders who want to see improvements. This often results in a piecemeal and chaotic approach, with a tendency for managers to be reactive rather than proactive.

It is the proactive providers and leaders, those who know the strengths and areas that are in need of improvement, who are most likely to actually see improved outcomes. That feels very obvious, and yet still I have seen even very large providers who are unaware of serious shortcomings because they have never looked. Instead, they focus on the 'swinging from the chandeliers' stuff – the high-profile innovation and seemingly cutting-edge initiatives that make for good newsletter content, but which fail to ensure that everyone is receiving safe care.

I recall the provider of a large teaching Trust asking to meet with me, in my capacity as the inspection lead and the chief inspector of hospitals, because they were both surprised and horrified that they had been downgraded to 'Requires Improvement'. They came armed with examples of their research, details of their newly opened immunity and transplantation centre, the profile of their board members (who had very impressive CVs) and their international work. They were indeed at the top of their field in some aspects of the treatment they provided. Unfortunately, they were also a little complacent about the everyday safe care and treatment of people using the service.

The Trust in question has more than eight hundred beds and serves a very large and mixed population. On three days, I walked around one of the hospitals and saw toxic cleaning fluid sitting on top of cleaning carts in the elderly care and children's wards. On the first day, I spoke to the then-Chief Nurse who said they would address the issue. On the second day, I did the same walk to see whether the situation persisted. Still, open and accessible cleaning fluids were on the same wards. I spoke with the Chief Nurse and asked whether they were aware of a recent death relating to the consumption of cleaning fluid in another NHS Trust. They were, and they agreed that it was shocking for an elderly patient to have died such a painful and avoidable death. I explained that there were still open bottles of toxic cleaning fluid (that could easily have passed as orange squash) on elderly care wards and a children's ward. They said they would address it – and by the way, could I tell them which wards it was on, please?

I suggested that they and a few matrons walked around to look at all wards where there were potentially vulnerable patients and to see for themselves how these things were being stored. I also suggested that rapid enforcement action and possibly an NMC referral might follow if the issue had not been addressed by the following day. In fairness, once the seriousness of the situation had been explained fully, the safety issue was addressed and the Chief Nurse came to find me the next morning with a completed audit of all wards across the Trust (which found far more wards with accessible cleaning fluid), orders for new cleaning carts with an easily closable and lockable compartment for toxic materials, and a requirement for all ward leaders to submit cleaning trolley visual compliance checks weekly.

The cleaning trolley issue was not the only reason for the downgrade, but it was certainly indicative of a board who had lost sight of the idea that safety is about the ordinary being done well, every day, rather than exceptional practice in small pockets of the service. It is about habitual good practice and providers knowing that this is happening. Providers and leaders in large services may well say that they "can't know everything about every aspect of a service", and to an extent this is true. Of course, a Chief Executive of one of the very large care home groups cannot know for certain that everyone with a heightened risk of pressure damage has their needs relating to skin integrity assessed, and their care plan delivered. They can, however, ensure that the systems that they have established make it easier for staff to provide good care, and that those staff enjoy providing safe care. They can ensure their governance processes provide assurance rather than reassurance. They can ensure that they resource services in a way that supports safe, high-quality care. And, most importantly, they can know the services they provide and understand where the risks are, what mitigations have been put in place, and how effective those mitigations are.

Governance of risk and safety is not just about seeing numbers on a screen. Governance at board level is not just about accepting reports as an accurate reflection of the service. It is a circle of knowledge-sharing that should be owned by everyone in a service. At its crudest, if an inspector can spot increased risk or poor practice, then the providers should have been a step ahead and should already have addressed it. Inspection teams do not have magic powers; they see what providers and registered managers could easily see for themselves if they only chose to look with an open mind.

Perceiving risks and shortcomings

There are all sorts of strategies and tools to help providers or registered managers know their service better. this. I would suggest that you begin when you accept a post, or when you set up or take over a service. What a wise leader will do is not assume that an initial look at the facts and figures is sufficient to ensure safety. Do look at the facts and figures, certainly, but don't assume they are the full picture. Likewise, don't assume that it is easier for a small provider to know how safe their service is and what the quality of care is; they have their own challenges that may obscure the picture. Few of us, after all, want to think the service we provide isn't good enough, and few health and care professionals entered their careers wanting to cause harm or injury. Why, then, do we not see the risks and shortcomings that inspection teams see?

I know when I became pregnant for the first time, there were suddenly huge bumps and tiny babies everywhere. When we bought an ancient Volkswagen Campervan to amuse our foster children, there were suddenly lots of people honking and waving at us from their similar vans on the roads of southern England. Had there been an unexplained rush to acquire a rusty split-screen or Type Two with an air-cooled engine? I think not. I'd just started noticing them as they had become relevant to me; a way of amusing children (and our cat – but that is another story) on our slow journeys to campsites.

Every second we receive countless bits of information in the things we hear, see, smell, touch and taste. We don't always register what this everyday information is or assimilate it fully. My husband has just put a coffee down beside me and gone out with the dog. I didn't hear or smell him making it, despite being in the same room as the coffee machine. We filter around two million bits of information per second. That is too much for us to actively process. For efficiency purposes, our brain has learned to filter out information that we don't need at that time. Some is archived for later use, some is dismissed, and some isn't even recognised as information. I didn't recognise the coffee-making as real information that needed processing.[19]

We usually focus on a handful of critical details at any given time. How many of us have been focused on whether there will be a parking space at the station and not noticed the speed we are travelling at on a country road? How many women have focused on their smudged eyeliner just before a meeting and not noticed that their dress is tucked into their knickers? We simply screen out seemingly unimportant information – and that includes the everyday things we see day in, day out.

The brains of an inspection team are trained to see things anew, to focus on risks and to observe things. They will inevitably see things that those

---

19 Csikszentmihalyi M (1990) *Flow: The psychology of optimal experience*. Harper Perennial.

working daily in a service don't see. Our experiences often act as an inadvertent screening tool and filter out low-probability risk, which is the opposite of commonsense risk. Everyone will still be able to see that leaving a used needle on a table in a children's ward playroom is a high risk, so would be likely to take action to address that risk. However, if a risk has a 1:1000 chance of being realised, then it is perceived as being unlikely to occur and may be dismissed. In regulated services, that may be cardboard boxes stored in the space under the stairs, or an external door to a postnatal ward fixed open in hot weather. Both situations require other things to happen before the risk is realised and an incident occurs, whether that be something to ignite the combustible material or someone wanting to take, or harm, a newborn infant.

These low-risk issues can easily escape our focus, especially if safety is falsely defined and measured by lack of accidents. Being exposed to risks multiple times without resulting in a poor outcome often results in our brains filtering it out. We are tricked into believing that we are safe. This can lead to dangerous complacency, where someone feels secure because they have stopped seeing potential dangers. When inspecting, I have often sat and observed in regulated services, finding a quiet corner where I am not in the way to just watch and listen. Initially, people are very aware that they are 'on show' and put on their best behaviours. After about twenty minutes, though, you become invisible. That is true of care homes, hospital wards, operating theatres, private hospitals, emergency department waiting rooms, GP waiting rooms... everywhere.

Once the veil of invisibility has descended, more usual and authentic practice can be seen. Often that is actually better behaviours, when staff are less nervous and not trying to be perfect professionals. In care homes and on elderly care wards, it might mean that people get more hugs, a member of staff sings 'Michael Row the Boat Ashore', someone living with dementia is calmed with an extra sugar in their tea, or a hot water bottle is offered to a woman with abdominal cramping on a gynae ward. Some of my most privileged work moments have been seeing the unguarded excellence that prevails in many services.

At the other extreme, where the culture is very different and not focused on excellence, the invisible inspector can quickly spot risks and safety shortcomings. Whether that be writing on fluid charts when no fluids have been consumed, not handwashing between supporting surgical patients, or removing walking aids to discourage people from walking around, staff quickly return to usual practice. Wise providers who really want to focus on ensuring they offer safe, high-quality care can use the device of invisibility to assist in the assessment of their service.

The psychology of observation and conversation

Observing is more than a brisk walk-around. Observation needs a clear purpose and focus to produce useful information. Observation does not always need to be done by the provider or executives, although if they take part in a planned programme of observation it may send a useful message about the importance of safety and quality. Often when I have led inspections of large Trusts, I am offered a record of visits by executives and non-executives. These may just be times and locations, or they may be more structured records with a box to tick about having spoken to staff, spoken to patients, and walked around a department. That has its place for ensuring senior visibility and making staff feel valued, but it doesn't do much to support safety.

Unsurprisingly, the psychology of board members works in a remarkably similar way to that of the rest of us. Research shows that people are more likely to talk to you if you are smiling. People are 86% more likely to strike up conversations with strangers in the street if they are smiling. We are naturally drawn to people who smile; negative facial expressions like frowns and scowls work in the opposite way, pushing people away.[20] If, as someone intent on speaking to staff and people using a service, you follow psychological norms, you will approach and initiate conversation with people who are smiling and making eye contact. That makes for a pleasant experience, but it is unlikely to identify service shortfalls. The person in the corner who smiles at staff is likely to get more staff attention; staff are likely to stop and chat while taking longer to help them with their medication. More attention may well result in fewer errors. The board member who speaks to smiling patients probably won't hear about being forgotten in the chaos of bed moves and not having had anything to eat that day.

Those services that use executive and non-executive walk-arounds might get a better picture by asking those board members to sit in the staff room at an ambulance station, or to sit in a bay on the acute medical unit and simply watch and listen.

A newly appointed registered manager will get a lot of information by speaking to staff. That information, however, may not be entirely accurate. People will be establishing relationships, may want to curry favour, or may want to be seen as a fount of all knowledge. They may want to maintain the status quo of less-than-ideal practice. Information obtained through conversation is usually opinion, which has some validity around the wider culture but is not necessarily relevant to the governance of safety. Sitting

---

20 Little AC, Jones BC & DeBruine LM (2011) Facial attractiveness: Evolutionary based research. *Philos Trans R Soc B.* **366** (1571) 1638-1659. doi:10.1098/rstb.2010.0404.

and watching how a medicine round is conducted may tell the new manager more about safe practice.

In my book *Towards Outstanding: Enabling Excellence in Care Home Provision* there are resources to complete a full assessment of the quality and safety of care homes.[21] The book goes on to offer a framework for quality improvement, but stresses that it can only be effective if it is based on a proper understanding of performance at the start. While focused primarily on care homes, the book is also useful and easily adapted to many other smaller services or parts of larger services. An independent healthcare company setting up an urgent treatment centre offering services in a very specialised setting recently used it to begin identifying areas they need to address as part of a registration process. For them, walking aids are unlikely to need to be considered, but the safe procurement, storage and administration of medicines will have much in common with care home medicines and will require the development of similar audit trails, with the involvement of a pharmacist. The consideration of good safeguarding practice needs similar thinking whatever the type of service.

Data and reports

As well as observation, services need to collate and review data around different aspects of safety. If there are no audits of records, no consideration of the number and themes of incidents reported, and no proper assessment of the numbers and skills mix of staff, then it will be hard to demonstrate that a service, however small, is safe. One of the first things a new registered manager or service leader should perhaps do is work through the paperwork related to their statutory safety obligations. It is possible to rely on external third-party contractors for aspects of care provision, but that does not negate the legal responsibilities of providers, managers or care professionals leading parts of services. A registered nurse manager in a psychiatric hospital might well face professional censure if a patient is injured in a fall from a window that they knew to be unrestricted. There is no option to say, "But estates is done by Another Company Ltd". In this scenario, the registered manager and provider might well face prosecution.

Do a proper assessment of third-party contracts and service-level agreements and how well they are being monitored. It's bureaucratic, and it probably isn't what you entered health or social care to do, but having accepted leadership responsibilities you cannot ignore them. You have chosen to be responsible for delivering safe care to service users, and that means ensuring that electrical equipment is tested and safe, that fire-safety systems are tested, working and safe, that windows have restrictors on them if necessary,

---

21   Salt T (2021) *Towards Outstanding: Enabling excellence in care home provision*. Pavilion Publishing and Media.

and that medical gases are stored properly. What did the last environmental health food hygiene report say? Are there contracts for equipment maintenance and are they providing a good service? A faulty hoist or sluice macerator presents significant safety risks.

It is easy to dismiss oversight of contracts as just bureaucracy until one looks at the personal costs; they are far more compelling than any CQC report could hope to be. In 2015, a healthcare firm and its director were ordered to pay more than £335,000 in fines and costs (closer to half a million now) because of a failure to provide safe care. The human cost was higher still. A 100-year-old resident died from injuries sustained in a fall from a hoist. The sling used to move her was very complicated to fit correctly, and the carers were given no training in how to safely use it. This led to the resident not being securely positioned within the sling, and, when she moved herself forward, she fell out, hitting the floor. Not a good way to die, and horrid for her relatives and the inexperienced care staff involved.

The centenarian's death could have been prevented had a better system for handling and moving residents, supported by appropriate staff training, been in place. Prior to this incident, another resident had fallen while being moved from her wheelchair to her armchair, breaking her tibia and fibula. Had someone running the home looked at the service-level agreement and hoist procurement, and looked at the training records, they might well have noticed and put together the previous accidents, the unsuitability of the equipment and the very limited training provided by the contract. The care home has now closed.[22]

The other very obvious thing to do when you have responsibility for the safety of a service is to look at the latest CQC report. Particularly look at the section detailing the 'shoulds' and 'musts'. These are very brief summaries of concerns identified. They don't offer the full evidential basis for determining care shortfalls or breaches of regulation, but they need to have been fully and sustainably addressed before the next inspection in order to avoid escalation of enforcement activity. If a service is currently rated 'Requires Improvement' or 'Inadequate' for safety, then the reasons for that need to be fully understood and there needs to have been sufficient action taken, with evidence of those improvements along with ongoing governance to ensure that people are safe. Some of the issues might seem a bit 'nit-picky' – but they are usually the quick wins, and so are easily addressed.

Personally, I get irritated if there is a focus on drug-fridge temperatures and records not showing the temperature of the fridge for a couple of days, particularly when the fridge has an automatic monitoring system

---

22 Applebey L (2015) *Care home owner sentenced after elderly resident dies falling from hoist* [online]. SHP. Available at: www.shponline.co.uk/common-workplace-hazards/care home-owner-sentenced-elderly-resident-dies-falling-hoist/ (accessed August 2023).

and especially if the report presented for quality assurance fails to identify whether pressure damage prevention measures are being used in line with planned care. I know that there is a theoretical risk of some drugs being rendered less effective if not stored at the correct temperature for a prolonged period of time, but I don't see fridge temperature as a thing that should be at the top of any risk consideration. That said, it will most likely be checked, and it is something that can be done very easily.

Why providers do not ensure that the basic things they know will be checked (like fridge-temperature monitoring) are completed properly is beyond me. I have heard many excuses over the years – "we're too busy", "it isn't a priority", "we're short-staffed" – but it is such a simple thing to get right, if you ask the right person and explain why it is important. If you expect an emergency nurse practitioner in a busy trauma centre to do it, it most likely won't get done until an inspector spots it and a requirement notice is issued. If you ask a clinical shift leader in a large nursing home caring for people living with dementia, it probably won't happen. If, however, you ask someone who wants more responsibility and to feel more involved as part of the ward team, then they will generally deliver daily checks every day. It doesn't need to be a registered nurse or pharmacist who checks that a fridge temperature has been recorded; if I was a senior leader in an NHS Trust, I might think about recruiting retired healthcare professionals to work with the pharmacy team to carry out such checks. They could go around the hospital, in an environment in which they felt comfortable, and tick all the fridge temperatures, thereby relieving staff of another job while ensuring medicines were stored at optimal temperature. Getting the jobs done sometimes requires focusing on outputs, and thinking outside the box.

In any setting, environmental checks to identify potential hazards don't have to be done by the manager. Of course, there are statutory environment and equipment checks that need professionally qualified people to carry them out through a formal contractual arrangement, but walk-arounds for spot checks are supplementary to these. Clearly, you don't want to pick someone off the street; there is a need to ensure that people are protected from inadvertent or deliberate harm, but volunteers can be properly recruited and trained to walk around, observe, and report back. Likely sources are people from the patient participation group of a GP practice, the relatives of someone who lived and died in a care home who want some legitimate way of continuing contact, or, in an acute hospital, a specific volunteer role could be created. There must be recruitment checks and oversight – there needs to be an agreed template and process with very clear limits to the role – but sometimes fresh eyes are better at spotting the worn carpet, the broken lavatory seats, the mouse droppings in the dining room or the scalding water in the basin in the staff changing rooms.

It can, of course, be non-executive directors, managers from other homes within a group or GP partners. It doesn't actually matter who goes around the premises (inside and out) and looks specifically for potential hazards. What matters is that someone does, that they report on this, and that their reports feed into a governance process that allows escalation of risks and action to reduce the risks. Someone mentioning a broken lavatory seat may prevent a fractured neck or femur. Someone mentioning a broken light bulb might prevent a fall. In different settings, the hazards might be different, so the walk-around might need to look at different things.

An ongoing process

Understanding a service is ongoing. Good safety governance requires assessment, risk identification, risk-reduction measures and monitoring through re-assessment. Part of that is the direct observation, the walk-arounds, the speaking with people using the service and staff, but the other critical part is collecting and understanding data. If you want to demonstrate that your service (or part of a service) is exceptionally safe, then you need to be able to produce the facts and figures to show that. In many services, producing the figures is easy – some data is available to inspection teams without needing to ask the service for it. Some is routinely collected and a statutory requirement through NHS commissioning, and some is required for benchmarking and performance oversight by larger corporate providers. But having the data is not sufficient – it needs to show that the service is performing well, improving against its own performance over time and outperforming its comparators. That is a bigger ask.

For small services, it is much harder but still essential to ensure that outcomes are consistently good and that there is a commitment to continuous improvement. In terms of ratings, most clinical audit data sits under the 'effective' rather than 'safe' key question. Most personal risk assessment data sits under the 'effective' key question, too – which is a bit of a change from the previous frameworks. That doesn't mean you can ignore the data around outcomes when trying to improve the rating for 'safe', as the two key questions are intrinsically linked. If staffing is low and the skills mix has seen a reduction in the ratio of registered nurses to support workers, then there are likely to be worse clinical outcomes. Conversely, if data around mortality, serious incidents or falls shows worsening outcomes, the leaders should be looking at their measures for the 'safe' key question to understand causality. It would be very difficult to claim a service was safe if the data showed that it was a mortality outlier, or if people using the service had an unusually high number of falls resulting in harm.

No single aspect of a service can really be considered in isolation. In order to be confident that they are offering safe care and treatment, providers and leaders need to understand their service well, and respond appropriately to reduce heightened risks.

Chapter 5: Building a culture of safety

I am sometimes asked: "How easy is it to get an 'Outstanding' rating for the 'safe' key question?" The answer is: it's hard. Very hard.

The 'safe' key question very rarely receives an 'Outstanding' rating. The reasons are multifactorial and not necessarily about the provider doing anything wrong. There are some overarching considerations that make it more likely, and that reduce the risk of a lower rating for the 'safe' domain – which would then limit the overall rating.

Across all service types and all core services, only about 4-5% of ratings are 'Outstanding'. At the other end of the scale, about 1-2% receive 'Inadequate' ratings. Most fall into the 'Good' rating category. When considering just the 'safe' key question, the ratings follow the same pattern, but fewer services get an 'Outstanding' rating and more get a 'Requires Improvement' rating.

A low rating for the 'safe' key question usually limits the overall rating. There is a possibility of an operational director and quality assurance panel stepping outside of the usual aggregation rules, but that is a rare occurrence. Generally, if you are given an 'Inadequate' rating for the safe domain, then your maximum overall rating will be limited to 'Requires Improvement'. Any breaches of regulation will limit the overall rating to 'Requires Improvement', at best. This is important to understand if you are aiming for an overall 'Outstanding' rating. It is worth spending time understanding the aggregation rules and how they feed into the overall ratings. They are available on the Commission's website.[23] For adult social care services, at least two of the five key questions would normally need to be rated as 'Outstanding', with the other three questions rated as 'Good', before an aggregated rating of 'Outstanding' could be given. There are a number of ratings combinations that will lead to a rating of 'Good'. The overall rating will normally be 'Good' if there are no key question ratings of 'Inadequate' and no more than one key question rating of 'Requires Improvement'.

It is all worked out using an aggregation tool; the rules are relatively simple for small services but the bigger the service, the more complex the aggregation becomes. A large NHS Trust may well have five key questions ratings for four core services across three sites, plus a 'well-led' question rating. This means that more than sixty individual ratings are being fed into the overall judgement. The rules can appear complex, but they feed

---

23 www.cqc.org.uk/guidance-providers/adult-social-care/how-we-aggregate-ratings-using-rating-principles-adult-social (accessed August 2023).

upwards rather than all sixty being lumped together to determine the final overall rating. The key question ratings give the core service rating. The core service ratings are aggregated to give the location rating, and the location ratings are aggregated to give the overall provider rating. The impact of one lower rating may be less obvious, although limiters still apply, so if one location has three 'Inadequate' core services then the overall rating is unlikely to be 'Good'.

Scoring and ratings

A scoring system is being introduced to improve the consistency of judgements, and to make the ratings system fairer and a more accurate reflection of the quality of a service. The four ratings of 'Outstanding', 'Good', 'Requires Improvement' and 'Inadequate' will remain as the changes to the methodology are introduced and embedded. There is no 'Satisfactory' rating as services are either good enough ('Good') or they need to improve in some way ('Requires Improvement'). Clearly, all services can and should continue to improve, but the ratings relate specifically to the regulations and whether or not a provider is meeting them.

Different Quality Statements are likely to be assessed over time and in different ways, as the CQC moves away from inspecting and reporting about a snapshot in time. Following an assessment, the evidence-scoring framework will be used, which should offer a more consistent and transparent view of quality and safety for people using all types of services. It should be less dependent on personal judgement and unconscious (or conscious) bias.

The evidence used to monitor and maintain the judgement around each service consists of an analysis of information held by the Commission. The amount and type of information held will vary depending on service type, but will include statutory notifications, results of national audits or surveys, mortality data, patient-safety incident data, safeguarding concerns about the service, whether there is a registered manager, the regulatory history and how the provider has responded and information from other stakeholders. This ongoing data analysis and monitoring sits alongside any inspection or remote Direct Monitoring Assessment activity. The evidence is used to determine the score for each Quality Statement:

4 = Evidence shows an exceptional standard of care

3 = Evidence shows a good standard of care

2 = Evidence shows shortfalls in the standard of care

1 = Evidence shows significant shortfalls in the standard of care

The Quality Statements clearly describe the standards of care that people should expect. Providers can improve their scores by ensuring that they can evidence that high-quality care, and that treatment is delivered in line with each Quality Statement. Additionally, there needs to be evidence covering each evidence category, and this guides the wise provider when deciding what to share via the portal or on inspection.

Scores for different Quality Statements will be updated at different times, leading to a more current and up-to-date view of quality. This may lead to changes in your rating. To make its judgement, the CQC will:

- Review evidence types within the required evidence categories for each Quality Statement.

- Apply a score to each of these evidence categories.

- Combine these required evidence category scores to give a score for the related Quality Statement.

- Combine the Quality Statement scores to give a total score for the relevant key question.

This score generates a rating for each key question, and aggregating the key question ratings gives the overall rating.

Ratings will be the only thing published initially, following introduction of the single assessment framework. It is likely that scores will published in the future, allowing people choosing or using services to understand the nature of the service more easily. Once the new scoring system is implemented, providers should be able to see how the judgement has been reached. The scoring system will show whether the quality of care is moving up or down within a rating, and it may give an indication that closer monitoring is needed.

Every service provider should aim for an 'Outstanding' rating and should take steps to ensure they are rated as at least 'Good'. Clearly, if there are no shortcomings in the care and treatment that people receive, then it will not be possible to give a lower rating following an inspection. If you aim for 'Outstanding' and don't quite make it, then you are still providing a good service. Complacency that accepts a low-scored 'Good' rating runs the risk of a breach of regulation or tipping into a 'Requires Improvement' rating. A 'Good' rating simply means that the Fundamental Standards are being met consistently – and by extension, wherever the standards are being met, the judgement should be for a 'Good' rating.

Why is there such variation and inconsistency across key questions when, in theory, they all carry the same weight? Well, there are many reasons why it is harder to get an 'Outstanding' rating in the safe domain than elsewhere.

Some relate to the process, some relate to the focus of an inspection team, some are about the inspection team's confidence and experience, and some are about how well the service has prepared for inspection. Hopefully, once embedded, the new scoring system and single assessment framework will go some way to improve how regulation is perceived.

A safety culture

The dominant culture within a health or social care service can have just as much impact on safety outcomes as the provider's safety-management systems. Really? Yes, really. It is not enough to have a system and the resources if they are not used effectively by people using the service and staff. Fire-safety doors only hold back fire if they are not wedged open! A poor safety culture has contributed to many major incidents, deaths and personal injuries. But what is a 'safety culture'? Well, it is about what is actually done in the workplace, rather than what the guidance, policy and regulations say *should* be done. A culture of safety is the mixing of staff, visitor and service user attitudes, shared values and perceptions that combine to form the 'how'.

I learned at a relatively early stage in my leadership career about the importance of a safety culture. I had line-management responsibility for a short-term children's home that had a very poor culture when I started in my role. The incumbent staff group and manager felt that they were 'listening to the young people' and building trusting relationships. In reality, this meant allowing smoking and drinking alcohol inside the building throughout the day. School was not seen as relevant, as the young people 'needed to talk', so entering the home almost needed breathing apparatus. The walls were yellowed and children as young as thirteen were lying around watching daytime television, drinking cider, smoking cigarettes purchased by staff and eating junk.

The second visit I made was to hold a meeting to tell the staff that policy and practice were changing. My vision was children attending school, staff taking the children shopping rather than doing bulk orders from the county suppliers, cooking proper meals from scratch, and introducing a range of constructive activities. I clearly didn't sell the message well enough, and I hadn't understood the potential risk of such a negative culture where poor practice was embedded. Shortly after I started in my new role, I received a call at two o'clock in the morning. I thought it was a hoax call, but no, there were eleven young people causing chaos at the local hospital. They had all been admitted with smoke inhalation problems because the home had burned almost to the ground. Luckily, nobody was seriously hurt and the two staff on duty overnight had managed to evacuate everyone.

After leaving the hospital, I arrived at a charred building and a large group of press. The staff had felt that I was a bit hard in stopping smoking completely and had 'turned a blind eye' to smoking that was not in communal areas. A fifteen-year-old lad had arrived back drunk and decided to smoke in bed. It could have been catastrophic. The root cause was the staff choosing to ignore policies and practices that were put in place to keep themselves and the children safe. They lost their jobs, but it was a small price to pay – they could have lost their lives.

A better-known example which highlights the inherent serious risks of a poor safety culture happened in January 2012. An Italian cruise ship, the Costa Concordia, capsized just off the coast of an Italian island in relatively shallow waters. The avoidable disaster killed thirty-two people and seriously injured many others. There are international maritime laws, company policies and safe operating procedures for sea-going vessels, but the habit of sailing close to shore to give passengers a nice view or salute other ships – a 'sail-by' – is not uncommon practice. They are a deviation from planned routes, a human decision by the captain or officers. Some consider them to be dangerous deviations. The investigative report found that the Concordia "was sailing too close to the coastline, in a poorly lit shore area, at an unsafe distance in the dark and at high speed." Safety was not the primary consideration of the captain, who was more focused on trying to impress a dancer.

Own and learn from mistakes

The example of the loss of the Costa Concordia was worsened by the crew trying to minimise the incident. The impact and water leakage caused an electrical blackout on the ship. Evidence discovered during the investigation showed that senior crew members had tried to downplay and cover up their actions, suggesting that a blackout was what actually caused the accident. This lack of honesty delayed the rescue and possibly added to the loss of life. It was over half an hour before the captain contacted rescue officials – the first call for assistance came from someone on the island. Somehow, the captain also made it to the lifeboat before many of his passengers, but he was sent back to his post. He was sentenced to sixteen years in prison.

The Commission publishes a few examples of learning from safety incidents and mistakes on their website.[24] The examples show the cost of failing to learn to the provider, the manager and for people using services. One such example is a care home provider and the registered manager who were prosecuted for failing to protect a resident from avoidable harm. A man had been a resident at the home since 2018. Three months after his admission, a social worker spoke to the registered manager and told her that the man was on the sex offender's register. Subsequently, the man sexually assaulted an elderly resident with dementia. Police were called

---

24   www.cqc.org.uk/guidance-providers/learning-safety-incidents (accessed August 2023).

and the man was arrested and later convicted. The court found that both the provider and the registered manager had failed to take all reasonable steps to protect people.

The court ordered the registered provider to pay a £128,000 fine and costs of £10,645 with a victim surcharge of £120. The registered manager was ordered to pay a £1,000 fine, costs of £15,067 and a victim surcharge of £100. Both provider and manager could have avoided the damage to their finances, and the manager could have avoided the loss of her job and the undoubted personal stress this caused, if only there had been a 'think safety' culture and an openness to learn from incidents. More importantly, the harm caused by a sexual assault on an elderly woman could have been avoided. A social worker informing a home that a resident is a known sex offender is an incident worthy of proper consideration from a risk perspective.

Listen

If only we/they had listened...

In April 2017 Ian Paterson, a surgeon working in the Midlands, was convicted of wounding with intent, and imprisoned.[25] He had harmed many patients in his care. The scale of his malpractice was shocking and the consequences tragic.

Paterson was trained as a general surgeon and also as a specialist breast surgeon in the NHS and independent sectors. There had been concerns about his surgical practice over many years. Other surgeons first raised serious doubts about his procedures and practice in 2003. He was convicted of seventeen counts of wounding with intent and three counts of unlawful wounding relating to nine women and one man treated as private patients between 1997 and 2011 and sent to prison for fifteen years. His jail sentence was felt to be too lenient and was increased by the Court of Appeal to twenty years. The national inquiry spoke with many patients – too many to quote here, but one account offers a degree of the injury Paterson caused:

"Patient 98 had some bleeding from her nipple and was referred to Solihull Hospital by her GP. She had a mammogram followed by an ultrasound and was told by Paterson the same afternoon that she had cancer in both breasts and needed to have her milk ducts removed urgently. He told her that there was a three-week wait in the NHS. Patient 98 had health insurance which covered limited procedures and decided to have surgery as a private patient at Parkway Hospital. Patient 98 saw Paterson regularly for three years after surgery, at which point he discharged her saying 'he had cured her of all the cancer'. Patient 98 found the period of time she was

25 https://assets.publishing.service.gov.uk/government/uploads/system/uploads/attachment_data/file/863211/issues-raised-by-paterson-independent-inquiry-report-web-accessible.pdf (accessed August 2023).

seeing Paterson very worrying and was concerned the cancer would return. She said her family was devastated, particularly her daughter who thought she would lose her Mum. Each time she saw Paterson she self-funded the consultation, ultrasound, and mammogram. She recalls on one occasion being charged £10 for the remaining strip of plaster he had used on her surgery wounds. Patient 98 was recalled by Spire. She was told that she had not had cancer and that her surgery had not been necessary."

In some cases, the treatment Paterson provided was not accepted practice, including the so-called cleavage sparing mastectomy (CSM). Patients had incomplete mastectomies without realising it. Paterson also failed on some occasions to complete full diagnostic tests. In other cases, surgical treatments and diagnostic tests were entirely unnecessary, and performed without any clinical justification. There were also accounts of patients having repeated surgeries and tests. In other cases, Paterson performed surgical procedures for which he was not qualified, some of which he was explicitly restricted from undertaking. We heard numerous concerns, from both patients and other witnesses, about the care provided by the breast-care nurse with whom Paterson worked in the private sector, and also the plastic surgeon with whom he worked very regularly in both the NHS and Spire.

Professionals raising concerns about a healthcare professional provides an opportunity to hospitals and others to examine the treatment and care that patients receive, and to stop any which is poor or inadequate. We heard that, in the case of Paterson, this did not happen in a way that was thorough or adequate. There were differences in how concerns were raised by professionals in the NHS and the independent sector. However, the response when professionals did raise concerns was inadequate in both sectors:

- The first concerns about Paterson were raised in 2003 by an oncologist who worked alongside him and was concerned that women were at increased risk of cancer recurring as a result of Paterson leaving tissue behind after surgery. The Trust's response to the investigation report was inadequate and placed patients at continuing risk of harm for a further seven years.

- In spring 2007, concerns about Paterson's conduct and clinical practice were raised by a newly appointed breast surgeon and two oncologists who worked alongside him. In response, Cunliffe, the Medical Director, and Goldman, the Chief Executive, set up an investigation under disciplinary procedures.

- In December 2007, six healthcare professionals who worked alongside Paterson were so worried about his clinical practice and patient safety that they wrote to the Chief Executive about him. The Trust investigated Paterson using HR processes, which meant that he was afforded confidentiality. This stood in the way of patient safety; patients being treated by Paterson were unaware that there were concerns about the safety of his operations.

- Many of the healthcare professionals who had raised concerns about Paterson were fearful of the consequences of doing so. Some had been reluctant to give evidence to the inquiry, and we believe that this was as a result of their negative experience of raising concerns.

- In the independent sector, raising concerns was similarly ineffective. Two local GPs who raised a concern about Paterson with a private hospital in 2008 claim they were told by the hospital manager in post at the time that he could not be suspended as he brought in too much income, although this was denied by the hospital director.

- Staff who raised concerns in the NHS assumed that their concerns were passed on; they were not. At the time, there were inadequate multi-disciplinary reviews, and Paterson was the only breast surgeon operating at the hospital. This may have contributed to his poor practice slipping under the radar and not being as apparent to others as it was in the NHS. However, when Paterson's patients were reviewed, the lead consultant said that, in his opinion, Paterson's malpractice should have been noticed by others. And yet none spoke up.

Make sure the evidence is provided

If an inspector observes that a member of staff signed a medicine chart for the wrong person, is it reasonable to say in a report that, "Staff did not always pay sufficient attention to the safe administration of medicine"?

There are lots of factors that come into consideration in this situation. Would that one observation make the comment valid if the service was a large Trust with over 1,500 beds? Would it be valid if the member of staff immediately realised their mistake and corrected it? Would it be valid if there was no harm from the incident and it was a recording error, rather than an administration error? Would it be valid if the service did not employ that member of staff – perhaps a community Trust staff member working in a polyclinic, or a GP making a home visit when a care home was being inspected?

The answer is to have the evidence available that demonstrates that medicines are managed safely. It is perhaps worth remembering that it is the provider or location that is inspected rather than individual staff members. Undoubtedly, in large and complex organisations, human factors mean that mistakes will happen. In regulatory terms, what is important is how the provider reduces the risks and takes measures to mitigate them. That is what needs evidencing.

Looking at the example above, where someone signs the incorrect medicine sheet, it would be very easy to say that no harm happened; to think that it is not *really* a problem, as it was corrected immediately. To an extent that is true – until the next time, that is, when a staff member not only picks up the wrong medicine charts but also uses it to give the wrong patient a high dose of an oral anticoagulant drug. That has potential consequences not only for Mr Kinnock who is now at increased risk of developing a serious blood clot but also for Mr Newell, who is at increased risk of falls and has bowel cancer.

What good providers do is provide evidence that they have safe systems for medicine management. That applies whatever the scale of the service and across all service types. They also show that they monitor how well the policies and protocols are followed across all areas of their service. They provide evidence of that monitoring over time – objective data and possibly observational audits of practice. They can demonstrate training and competency assessment and show how they react to incidents and errors. When an error or near miss occurs, it is not dismissed. Someone 'walks the journey' as part of a root cause analysis. Perhaps if someone had 'walked the journey' when the wrong medicine chart was signed, they might have realised that keeping all the medicine charts stacked on the drug trolley, in a pile that was accessed by numerous staff in a fast-paced assessment unit, was almost inviting a mistake. Would that error have been made if the charts were kept at the end of the beds?

Inspectors are not psychic. They can only write about the evidence they have. They can ask for it, of course, but far better it is given upfront and explained. So give them a file of evidence. Make their job easier.

Build a learning culture

I think many providers talk very well about building a safety culture, listening to staff and learning when things go wrong. Every regulated organisation has a policy. Every registered manager can talk about learning from mistakes. Yet for the reporting year to January 2023, there were 325 Serious Incidents reported which appeared to meet the definition of a 'Never Event' (an incident that should never happen if available preventative measures have been implemented). In the three-month period from April to June 2022, a total of 652,246 incidents were reported via the National Reporting and Learning System. While most caused little or no harm to people using services, it still suggests that lessons have not been learned, or that learning is not embedded.

Care home residents are three times more likely to fall than people living in the community, and they are ten times more likely to sustain a significant injury as a result.[26] Some of this is about the frailty of the people resident in a care home, but some is also avoidable harm. Around 40% of admissions from care homes to hospitals are related to falls.[27] A study of a multifactorial

---

26   Cooper R (2017) Reducing falls in a care home. *BMJ* 6 (1). Available at: https://bmjopenquality.bmj.com/content/6/1/u214186.w5626 (accessed August 2023).

27   Logan PA *et al* (2021) Multifactorial falls prevention programme compared with usual care in UK care homes for older people: multicentre cluster randomised controlled trial with economic evaluation. *BMJ*. Available at: www.bmj.com/content/375/bmj-2021-066991 (accessed August 2023).

falls prevention programme in UK care homes was associated with a reduction in fall rate and cost effectiveness, without a reduction in activity or increase in dependency. Falls can in many cases be prevented. It is about creating a mindful and reflective culture of safety rather than simply accepting that older people have falls.

NHS England has a national Patient Safety Strategy and says that patient safety is about maximising the things that go right and minimising the things that go wrong.[28] Their website suggests that safety is integral to the NHS's definition of quality in healthcare, alongside effectiveness and patient experience.

On the whole, children and young people have powerful advocates in their parents who are likely to be a very visible and possibly vocal presence on a children's ward. Paediatric staff are trained to work in partnership with parents and carers, and with the young people themselves. This helps to ensure that care is provided safely, in a timely way. That is not to say that things do not sometimes go horribly wrong. In June 2001, the government report *Learning from Bristol* was published. This was the Department of Health's response to the public inquiry into children's heart surgery at Bristol Royal Infirmary. Over a five-year period (1991-1995), thirty-four children under one year of age died at Bristol. It was believed that they would have survived in other NHS units.

In thinking about this, one must remember that this was a highly specialised tertiary service where the risks were always going to be high: the issues that resulted in avoidable deaths at Bristol have led to significant changes in regulation and reporting across the NHS. The report highlighted many problems that are a recurrent theme in the reports of national inquiries. It seems that, even after truly tragic events come to light, we don't always think the findings contain lessons for every healthcare service. The themes identified following the Bristol investigation mention "staff shortages, a lack of leadership, an 'old boy's culture' among doctors, a lax approach to safety, secrecy about doctors' performance and a lack of monitoring by management." One finding in particular is replicated time and again by investigations and through inspection processes. As early as 1991, one doctor raised concerns about mortality rates with Trust executives. He also contacted the NHS, the Department of Health, and the Royal Colleges. He was largely ignored until the tragic death of baby Joshua Loveday during a complex heart operation.

On October 9th, 2020, the CQC announced that it would be criminally prosecuting East Kent Hospitals NHS Trust on two counts of unsafe car and treatment for Harry and Sarah Richford. This was the first time in the UK that an NHS Trust had been prosecuted for unsafe clinical care. On

28 www.england.nhs.uk/patient-safety/the-nhs-patient-safety-strategy/ (accessed August 2023).

November 2nd, 2017, baby Harry Richford had been born on his due date at Queen Elizabeth the Queen Mother Hospital in Kent, following a healthy pregnancy. Everyone expected a normal birth and Sarah, his mother, was classified as low risk. Harry died seven days later following a botched labour, delivery and resuscitation.

The Trust entered a plea of guilty and was fined £733,000. Harry's father's statement to the coroner in January 2020 said, "I'm not just one voice, I am the voice for all those who have suffered at the hands of the Trust and their inadequate maternity department. We respectfully ask the coroner to consider the fact that it is the family's real wish to seek justice for all of those that have been in this position." Deepening the tragedy of Harry's death is the fact that in November 2015 an expert group reviewed the provision of obstetric and maternity services at the Trust. The report cited several issues and made a number of recommendations. The organisation had failed to learn, and the result was Harry's death.

Harry's grandfather suggested that we should "go into hospital with your eyes wide open". Those open eyes are particularly important for the staff and leaders of all services providing health and social care. While Harry's death is an immeasurable and unique pain for his family, I am sure it is also a deep pain for the healthcare professionals involved who must live with some degree of culpability. What is perhaps most concerning is that it is not the first time there have been concerns that have resulted in the death of babies. Not the first time that there has been a lack of openness and transparency, and not the first time that parents have tried to raise concerns about poor maternity and obstetric care.

Many people who complain about unsafe healthcare don't want financial compensation; they want to stop others feeling the same pain. They want to prevent further tragedies and make care and treatment safer for others. In 2008, baby Joshua Titcombe died at nine days old. His father had to campaign long and hard to be listened to. Records were said to be lost. Concerns were dismissed. Five-and-a-half years later, in March 2015, the Kirkup report was published. It described a dysfunctional maternity team within University Hospitals of Morecambe Bay NHS Trust, where certain midwives were reluctant to seek medical assistance because of their commitment to a 'normal birth'. Relationships between doctors and midwives were poor, and midwifery practice fell well below acceptable standards. Importantly, instances of avoidable harm and death were covered up. Lessons were not learned, and mistakes were repeated year after year. The report detailed how opportunities to intervene were missed at all levels, and how the families who raised concerns were treated as problems to be managed, rather than voices that needed to be heard.

Move forward to 2022, when the Ockenden Report was published, and we find another Trust where the story sounds somewhat familiar. The Independent Maternity Review of maternity services at the Shrewsbury and Telford Hospital NHS Trust looked into an NHS maternity service that failed. It failed to investigate, failed to learn, and failed to improve, and therefore often failed to safeguard mothers and their babies at a critical time in their lives. Twelve maternal deaths were reviewed. The team concluded that none of the mothers had received care in line with best practice at the time and, in three-quarters of cases, the care could have been significantly improved.

The executive summary says, "The internal investigations frequently did not recognise system and service-wide failings to follow appropriate procedures and guidance. As a result, significant omissions in care were not identified and, in some incidents, women themselves were also held responsible for the outcomes." It goes on to report that, "As part of the review, 498 cases of stillbirth were reviewed and graded. One in four cases were found to have significant or major concerns in maternity care that, if managed appropriately, might or would have resulted in a different outcome."

It would be easy to dismiss reports like those mentioned above as 'only being about maternity care' or 'only being about the NHS', but that is probably why we see history repeating itself. Serious safety and care failings can too easily be dismissed as being about other people, other places, other types of service. Learning from incidents is not just about learning from the mistakes and shortcomings in a particular service. An open and transparent culture that places people using the services centre stage would want to share its learning, surely?

Lessons have not yet been learned well enough.

Chapter 6: People make mistakes

In health and social care errors can have significant costs, both human and financial. Wrong site surgery, incorrect reading of CTGs during labour, driving too fast on blue lights across a busy junction, not reporting the torn carpet in a care home's corridor, dismissing the mother of a child with a rash as an overly worried parent... all these have the potential for tragedy. And all could be avoided. For this reason, when deciding on policy, carrying out investigations and reviews, or conducting public and professional discussions, human and moral factors must always be considered. We all make mistakes, and most of us learn from them – that is the very nature of maturing. Hopefully, most of our mistakes don't have devastating consequences and, if we reflect honestly, we can realise what factors contributed to them.

My own mistakes are too numerous to list, and I have definitely repeated some. Last week a letter arrived from Yorkshire Police asking who was driving my car at 82mph on a stretch of dual carriageway. This won't be the first speed-awareness course I have attended. It will cost me a little, and I will try to be more observant about average speed zones and mobile speed camera vans in future. Did I intend to get photographed in order to receive a fine and a morning in a grim hotel somewhere? No, of course not. The factors that came into play were entirely human, and that applies to each and every time I have been caught speeding.

Just to be clear, my last speeding course was around ten years ago. Generally, I like to think I am quite an observant and safe driver. I know the potential consequences of speeding and yet, like most of us, I still do it occasionally. I suppose I assume that on a fairly empty dual carriageway in good weather it's unlikely that I'll cause a problem. Except, of course, that the consequences of a crash increase significantly with speed. High-speed crashes are more likely to occur than crashes at lower speeds and, when they do occur, they're more likely to be deadly. At higher speeds, drivers have less time to brake or swerve, while vehicle braking distances increase. Research also shows that we are less aware of our peripheral vision at higher speeds and are less likely to see or predict potential dangers, such as pedestrians crossing the street or children playing. Crashes are more likely to kill at higher speeds, for the simple reason that they are more forceful.[29]

---

29 NACTO (2023) *Speed Kills* [online]. Available at: https://nacto.org/publication/city-limits/the-need/speed-kills/ (accessed August 2023).

I know all that, and I have been on a speed awareness course, yet I still sometimes speed – so clearly education isn't everything. To reduce speeding, there must be systems in place to encourage me to do the right thing and put my car's speed restrictor on. It cannot be left to personal choice and preferences, as some people (like me) won't follow the guidance. That's why those responsible for road safety need to understand why people speed, and put in place measures to reduce the risk. There are deterrents, but they aren't foolproof; I am convinced that the appearance of huge, deep, unrepaired potholes is a covert local-authority strategy not only to reduce road repair costs but also to reduce the number of road traffic accidents.

So why do I speed? And why did I get caught speeding? The two are not exactly the same thing, but they are related. On both occasions when I have been caught speeding, I have been offered a speed awareness course because I was speeding on a dual carriageway in good driving conditions. I had my music on and was singing along. The car is the only place where I am allowed to sing, and even then, the windows have to be shut. I'd got my cappuccino from a machine at the petrol station. And I was enjoying myself – but clearly, I wasn't really concentrating. Mistakes aren't always about being stressed or having insufficient resources. They are often about that very human state – distraction. None of us wants to be caught speeding, just as very few people want to give the wrong drug to someone.

Human rather than technical failures are possibly the biggest risk in complex and potentially hazardous systems. This includes health and social care organisations. Managing the human risks can never be one hundred percent effective. Human fallibility can be moderated, but it cannot be eliminated. In healthcare, eighty percent of errors are attributed to human factors at individual level, organisational level, or commonly both.[30] Understanding how human factors impact on care and treatment delivery and organisational policy can have a fundamental effect on patient safety.

Human factors encompass all those factors that can affect the behaviour and performance of people in a system. It allows us to understand how people perform under different circumstances and why mistakes happen. Here are some examples:

■ A hospital where the handwash basins deliver water at 47° Celsius cannot be surprised if an observational audit shows staff do not follow the NHS handwashing technique guidance and the incidence of infection rises. In this case, the provider is not making it easy for staff to wash their hands properly.

---

30 East Lancashire Hospitals NHS Trust (undated) *A Focus on Human Factors* [online]. Available at: www.elht.nhs.uk/application/files/5415/6346/2311/Share2Care_Human_Factors_FINAL_WEB_180119.pdf (accessed August 2023).

- If an anaesthetist is very late for the start of an operating list and the staff have put everything out ready, including syringes full of the drugs that are required, knowing that the surgeon will be shouting at them to hurry up, then it would hardly be surprising if the incorrect drug was handed to the anaesthetist.

- If a junior doctor is up all night covering the medical wards of a hospital, then has to stay on because the locum for the day shift has not arrived, it is hardly surprising if they write '10mg Oral Morphine hourly' rather than 'four-hourly'. If the nurse administering it is newly qualified, and the second checker is an agency nurse, then it is less likely to be picked up. Especially if the newly qualified nurse is worried because the ward sister is off sick, and the agency nurse is new to the hospital and working additional shifts to pay the rent.

It's not just in hospitals. If a GP telephones a care home and prescribes increased warfarin for Mr Thorn because his blood results indicate this is required, and the receptionist writes a note for the manager but loses it under a pile of paperwork and tells the nurse in charge of the shift that the doctor has said Mr Swan should double his warfarin dose, then Mr Swan and Mr Thorn are both placed at risk. The incident is about human factors, rushing, distraction and poor communication. It could, of course, be prevented by care home staff and the GP practice working together around effective communication pathways.

In late 2018, the CQC published a report called *Opening the Door to Change* which looked at the factors that contributed to the occurrence of 'Never Events' and serious patient-safety incidents. Between April 2017 and March 2018, there were 468 incidents classified as 'Never Events' in the UK. The report says that too many people are being injured or suffering unnecessary harm because NHS staff are not supported by sufficient training, particularly around human factors, and because the complexity of the current patient safety system makes it difficult for staff to ensure that safety is an integral part of everything they do. The findings also apply to those independent healthcare services that offer treatment to NHS patients.

Two examples of human factors in action

Example 1

Let's think of an example where a lack of consideration of human factors resulted in a series of 'Never Events' in a large, prestigious NHS Trust that expected to be rated 'Outstanding' (but wasn't). The Trust ran three acute hospitals, each with their own executive team. The Trust executives were not involved in the day-to-day running of the hospitals, but saw themselves as entirely strategic, outward facing and focused on developing system-wide protocols and pathways. They were doing some really innovative work and, undoubtedly within tertiary services, there were pockets of international renown and excellence. Unfortunately, that resulted in the three hospitals being managed in three different ways, with little organisation-wide learning.

The first series of five 'Never Events' related to patients who, requiring oxygen, were connected to an air rather than oxygen flowmeter. Most of these incidents did not result in apparent patient harm; in one case, however, the patient deteriorated rapidly and required critical care. In discussion with the board members nobody was aware of these incidents, and nobody had seen a trend as the incidents had occurred in the three different hospitals. The information hadn't been disseminated well, and nobody had considered the human factors or simple mitigations that could have prevented further incidents after the first was recorded. The local executives for each hospital didn't want their shortcomings publicised, possibly because they knew the Trust's Chief Executive role was being vacated shortly after the inspection. It was all kept in-house because of unnecessary competition rather than shared within a collaborative culture. It's only human to want to compete a bit, isn't it? Targets and dashboards between different sites or parts of an organisation often encourage that exact tendency.

The investigations into the incidents didn't consider human factors, and suggested the causality was that the 'Never Event' was newly introduced and not yet widely known, particularly among agency staff – so emails were sent to all staff reminding them. Nobody stopped and said that, even if this type of incident wasn't on the 'Never Event' list, it still shouldn't happen, and nobody asked why. A lack of skills and competency can be a human factor, but all the doctors and nurses who connected the tubing to the outlets on the wall would already be aware that it was oxygen that had been prescribed. They all knew the difference between three litres of oxygen per minute and air. It wasn't credible to consider this a lack of knowledge, yet the action plan was about training during team meetings on one site, email reminders on another, and an e-learning programme on the other. The investigations didn't consider staffing levels or acuity. There was no cross-organisation consideration of any common factors (four of the incidents occurred in emergency departments).

It was a wider issue than just the one NHS Trust. In 2021 (after the inspection of the Trust above, which took place in 2019) a national patient safety alert was circulated.[31] Over a three-year period from 2018 to 2021, 108 'Never Events' describing similar unintentional connections were reported. Over one-third of incidents occurred in emergency departments. Consequences included respiratory arrest, cardiac arrest, and collapse (requiring ITU admission and ventilation); six patients subsequently died.

---

31   www.england.nhs.uk/wp-content/uploads/2021/06/Air-flowmeter-NaPSA-FINAL.pdf (accessed August 2023).

A review of the 108 reported incidents indicated that misconnection was often an 'unconscious error' (i.e., the person does not realise that they have made a wrong connection) and so incidents often went undetected even when other staff responded to deterioration. The recommended solutions are very simple and seemingly obvious if one accepts that human factors in an emergency department might see staff acting under pressure, who are stressed and possibly fatigued. A gas outlet on the wall, with two almost identical flowmeters to connect oxygen tubing to, feels like a recipe for a mistake. We asked the provider why they had not capped the air outlet or replaced the dual flowmeter with a single one connected only to the oxygen. The answer was that the emergency department staff often needed to access the air outlet to run nebulisers. We asked why they didn't use compressor nebulisers that didn't need connecting to a gas outlet. We were told they hadn't got enough, and it was easier for staff to connect to air from the wall above the bed space than try to find a nebuliser that was decontaminated and ready to use.

That was a very clear example of a provider not making it easier for staff to do the right thing. By enabling this unsafe practice, it was not saving staff effort and time – it is much harder for staff to report an incident, be part of an investigation, apologise to patients or families and possibly attend a coroner's hearing or inquest. It was not saving the provider money; providing assurance to CQC and the commissioners and introducing yet more e-learning are expensive. Inspections in response to a potential trend of serious incidents cost a lot, and negligence claims cost a huge amount.

A comprehensive review with a willingness to consider human factors can improve learning from incidents and thus reduce patient harm. Using single gas flowmeters and capping air outlets in the emergency departments to make it easier to use one of the many compressor nebulisers purchased after the first 'Never Event' might well have been cheaper, certainly more pleasant and less time-consuming for staff, and definitely safer for patients.

Example 2

The second example comes from a care home provider that I worked with. They had a very people-centric culture and wanted to ensure everyone received safe care without restricting choices for individuals. They were very good homes with a comprehensive governance system and very interested provider. They understood that medicines errors could have serious consequences for people using the service, many of whom were living with dementia and would not have recognised an incorrect tablet being offered. They also understood that it was very easy for staff who were busy or agency staff who were unfamiliar with the home to make mistakes.

They invested in a system that made it easy to do the right thing. It allowed electronic ordering, dispensing, storage and administration, reducing the risk of medication errors. The access to medication was limited and only trained staff could administer drugs. Each person had a named box in the medicines trolley to store their prescribed medicines. Their medicines were dispensed in named containers by the pharmacist who oversaw the medicines management arrangements and carried out audits through a contractual arrangement. The drug storage room was temperature controlled to ensure that medicines remained effective. Access to the room was limited, and the person accessing could be identified through the electronic system with which they recorded the details of everyone who entered the room.

The records relating to medicines monitoring and audits and any medicines errors were reviewed by the head of quality and safety leads for the provider, and by the regional directors. There were robust governance arrangements and, where errors happened, comprehensive reviews were carried out and shared across all homes in the group. The heads of quality, regional directors and providers were known to home staff and people living at the home. They visited regularly and spoke to everyone they came across when walking around. They were visible and approachable, as were the registered managers. They had built a culture where staff enjoyed providing high-quality, safe care, and where people felt they could raise concerns.

Chapter 7: The 'Dirty Dozen' of human error

The 'Dirty Dozen' refers to twelve of the most common human error preconditions, or conditions that can act as precursors to incidents. These twelve elements influence people to make mistakes. The 'Dirty Dozen' is a concept developed by Gordon Dupont in 1993, while he was working for Transport Canada.[32] In fact, much of the work around human factors and safety systems comes from the aviation industry. One can imagine the devastation if safety precautions and checks are not followed when a large aeroplane is taking off, full of families heading on their holidays. The twelve factors are probably something we all recognise from times when we have reflected on mistakes we have made, or on those we have seen others make.

1. Communication

This includes both written and verbal communication. I remember when I was working a set of nights on a paediatric intensive care unit, calling through a barely opened door to an agency nurse asking them to give a baby some GEM (a gastro-electrolyte mixture that was prescribed to maintain the hydration of the tiny and very sick baby via a naso-gastric tube). Shortly afterwards, the ventilator alarms sounded, and I looked on in horror to see the agency nurse about to spoon strawberry jelly down the endo-tracheal tube. Luckily, they were stopped before any harm had come to the infant and the breathing tube was reconnected swiftly. Entirely down to poor communication and assumptions about a colleague's understanding.

2. Distraction

Who doesn't get distracted? The member of care staff who needs to collect his child from school and is running late? The paramedic waiting to hear about her son's exam results? The GP with pregnancy-related nausea? The surgeon waiting to hear the results of a biopsy? The registered nurse doing a drug round and being repeatedly interrupted by a stream of other staff?

Distractions such as these cannot be addressed by policy, but the risks can be mitigated in particularly high-risk settings, by ensuring consistent use of safety systems and by growing a culture where it is okay to tell others that you are a bit distracted because your elderly mother has just had a serious fall. The factors are inevitably entwined. An organisation with good teamworking will understand that their colleague is an only child, and that their mother lives an hour away. They will make accommodation for these

---

32 Skybrary (2023) *The Human Factors "Dirty Dozen"* [online]. Available at: https://skybrary. aero/articles/human-factors-dirty-dozen (August 2023).

circumstances. Of course, a good leader will already know that the staff member has remote caring responsibilities, and will perhaps have offered carer's leave so they can take time to go and ensure their mother is okay.

3. Lack of resources

Good care costs less. It really does. Where staffing levels are not sufficient to meet the needs of the people using the service, errors increase. Accidents increase. Outcomes worsen. Providers who invest in their people will see lower levels of serious safety incidents. Providers who ensure they resource their services properly will see fewer serious patient-safety incidents.

Caring for someone discharged to their care home following a fractured neck or femur will require more staff time to help them dress, to help them move, to address their pain and to reassure their relatives. There might be a complaint or a safeguarding investigation. The commissioners might want to understand how this person fell and was not found for three hours. That is all expensive, resource-heavy and demoralising for staff, as well as being very unpleasant for the person who was injured.

4. Stress

There are many types of stress. Some are about the here and now, and some have built up or have an impact over time. Nobody doubts that having to provide care and treatment at the site of a major disaster is stressful. It places demands on the senses, the emotions and the bodies of those working in such circumstances. Conversely, chronic stress accumulates and results from long-term, and often multiple, demands placed on staff. Some of the stressors may be work related – short staffing, long and unsocial hours. frequent shift changes, limited resourcing, and, of course, culture. Some may be outside of work but still have an impact on how people perform.

Stress, especially chronic stress, can change the way in which we react to everyday occurrences. Colleagues and managers may see the signs of stress emerging as changes in mood and personality, lack of judgement, lack of concentration and poor memory. If we are preoccupied with worrying about the electricity bill and our teenage daughter's friendship with a much older man, we may well not remember that an agency care worker wasn't able to give Mr Bryson his insulin. Long-term stress can make people more susceptible to infections, increased use of stimulants and self-medication, absence from work, illness and depression. People can also become irritable, and this is compounded by the effect of high doses of caffeine – when irritability and insomnia add to the stress symptoms. No provider wants staff to be off sick with stress, and no staff member wants to live with stress levels that have a significant impact on his or her wellbeing.

A wise provider will have known channels of communication available to signpost staff to options that can help them rationalise their concerns, in order to manage stress in positive ways that improve their health and to get any practical or financial help available. There are some very good resources out there, and a culture that supports rather than criticises goes a long way to enabling staff to manage their stress levels. Some of that is around fair recruitment of people who are able to manage the demands of the role they are being appointed to, some is about allowing staff to feel success, and some is about making adjustments that are a reasonable way of supporting staff beyond the requirements of the Equality Act 2010.

5. Complacency

Complacency is about thinking we are doing a job well, believing we know our subject thoroughly and being very comfortable with our performance at the same time as forgetting or dismissing risks. It's a belief that we are so competent that the risks become irrelevant, that it couldn't happen to us.

Complacency often arises when thinking is taken out of routine activities that have become habitual, and that may be thought of as easy and safe. Relaxing vigilance means important safety signals may be missed. People often only see what they expect to see. While high demand causes stress and reduced human performance, too little demand can result in boredom, complacency, and reduced performance. It is therefore important, when conducting simple, routine tasks repeatedly, to maintain an optimum level of stress through different stimulation. That doesn't mean trying to support someone to eat and drink while standing on a tightrope!

Many years ago, I worked with a service that provided care for girls with learning disabilities. We used to take a group swimming most weeks – an activity that was open to all. It was very popular and an easy activity for staff. The local swimming pool staff knew us well and were very welcoming. Long before I arrived, it was decided that any girl who had epilepsy would not be stopped from swimming but would be required to wear a yellow swimming hat. As everyone wore swimming hats, most were not aware of why they had been offered a specific colour. They were just handed out by the house staff who knew which girls needed a yellow hat.

The pool lifeguards were also made aware of the yellow hats. Their usual relaxed style of observation changed noticeably. While our girls were in the pool, they didn't sit at the end, leaning on the pool cover roll, chatting, but maintained a very engaged observation walking around the pool, ensuring someone was at the deep end and following the three or four yellow-hatted girls with eagle eyes. The house staff sitting in the spectators' gallery also followed the yellow-hatted girls as they swam freely around, diving, racing and giggling, and entirely unaware of any difference. Society wouldn't single people out with yellow hats now, but at the time it stopped complacency.

A modern healthcare-related example is the World Health Organization's 'Five Steps to Safer Surgery' checklists that are used in every hospital in the country that offers surgery. That is a visible and audible reminder to ensure that the correct operations are being carried out on the right people.

6. Lack of teamwork

In most services, tasks and care delivery are about teamwork. Rarely is a single person responsible for safe outcomes of a particular task. Even when we think an incident is about the actions or omissions of one person, a comprehensive consideration and reflection often show that there is wider responsibility.

Let's consider a situation in which someone is left in pain because the prescribed drug is not available. It might happen in a care home, in a hospital or in an ambulance – the type of service is irrelevant. Who is responsible for the pain that person is suffering? Is it acceptable to think that the patient using community healthcare services who forgot to order more from their GP is at fault? What if they have some form of cognitive impairment? Does the blame sit with their daughter, who is juggling work, elderly parents and teenage children and who lives over an hour away?

The staff member who administered the last dose or second-to-last dose of the drug should probably have ordered more, shouldn't they? The person who assessed the pain should probably have taken action to find some, or to get a different drug prescribed. They should certainly have used non-pharmaceutical methods to alleviate the pain. The responsible manager might want to consider whether they have sufficient oversight of medication. The prescriber might want to consider whether their prescription offered sufficient analgesic options. The pharmacist might want to ensure good stock control, prescribing and audit. They might also want to ensure that prescribers are aware of any potential shortages. The provider might want to think about their policy and processes for ensuring adequate pain relief. One might even question whether the government and national bodies have put in sufficient mitigation to reduce the risk of drug shortages.

Looking to apportion blame and scapegoat is not the way to ensure excellence in care delivery. Of course, people should be held to account for intentionally poor practice, but a helpful reflection will consider whether training and competency assessments are effective, whether policies are enacted (and if not, why not), whether staffing levels are appropriate, whether support is available to avoid incidents, and whether governance and interprofessional communication in effective.

If someone is not contributing to the team effort, this can lead to unsafe outcomes. We all have to rely on each other. In health and social care environments, we have to rely on many others and ensure we collaborate to provide good care and the right treatment. That means we need to work not only with our immediate team but also the wider organisational and external partners and agencies. Teamwork consists of many skills and levels of expertise that each team member brings, and when that is not valued and respected, the person receiving care is likely to have worse outcomes.

This is so important; I am going to labour the point:

Teams need to work together for the benefit of service users.

Some of the key teamwork skills required are around leadership, effective communication, trust, motivation, and recognition and valuing.

To create an effective team, there are a few pre-requisites and ongoing actions required. The risk of 'just allowing it to develop naturally' are high. It is entirely possible for a toxic culture to grow where there is a canyon created by poor leadership. It happens in large healthcare organisations, as national reports (such as the Ockenden Report and The Gosport Independent Panel Report) show.[33] It happens outside of healthcare, and one only needs to consider the Oxfam inquiry, the Baroness Casey Review of the culture of the Metropolitan Police to understand it is not about the type of organisation, nor is it confined to a few high-profile NHS Trusts.[34, 35]

There are numerous resources available that provide advice on growing a positive culture, on team building and on good leadership, so it is not my intent to detail those here. Each provider needs to understand the prevailing culture of their organisation and where there are pockets or teams that sit outside the core culture. That can work either way, of course. A generally happy and motivated NHS Trust might find a pocket of staff in a particular speciality who are demotivated, do not support changes to working practice, appoint 'people like us' and suppress challenges. The leaders at executive and middle-management levels need to work with the poorly performing team to bring them into the fold of collaborative working and patient-centric care.

Similarly, a provider with four care homes may find that one care home is excelling, while the others have high attrition rates, more complaints, higher staff sickness levels and more medicine errors. That provider would do well to understand what is different and share that learning with the homes providing a worse experience for staff and people using the service. It will be about leadership and poor team working, but the provider needs to understand fully what that means for each service.

---

33   www.gosportpanel.independent.gov.uk/ (accessed August 2023).

34   https://assets.publishing.service.gov.uk/government/uploads/system/uploads/attachment_data/file/807943/Inquiry_Report_summary_findings_and_conclusions_Oxfam.pdf (accessed August 2023).

35   www.met.police.uk/SysSiteAssets/media/downloads/met/about-us/baroness-casey-review/update-march-2023/baroness-casey-review-march-2023a.pdf (accessed August 2023).

7. Pressure

Pressure is inevitable when working in a dynamic and complex environment. Sometimes it helps us to deliver, but when the pressure to meet a deadline interferes with our ability to complete tasks correctly, it has become too much. Targets are a measure, and they should never be used as a battering ram on staff who are working hard to deliver in difficult circumstances. It is the old argument of quantity versus quality. In health and social care, we should never knowingly reduce the quality of our work.

Pressure can be created in all sorts of ways:

- by lack of resources, especially time
- by our own inability to cope with a situation
- by direct, or indirect, pressure from managers, people using services or colleagues.

One of the most common sources of pressure is ourselves. We put pressure on ourselves by taking on more work than we can handle, never learning to say no. In health and social care staff tend to be kind, and so may take on other people's problems. When deadlines are critical, extra resources and help should always be provided to ensure the task is completed to the required quality. There is little point keeping to a four-hour emergency department target if the pressure to meet this for over 95% of patients arriving means that they are discharged too quickly only to be readmitted four hours later. Decisions made under pressure may not be the right ones.

8. Situational awareness

Situational awareness is about a continuous process and perception of the elements in an environment, and a comprehension of their meaning and the importance of that ongoing information in the near future. This basic definition has been extended by Cindy Dominguez and colleagues, who stated that situational awareness needs to include the following four specific elements:[36]

- Extracting information from the environment – seeing, hearing, smelling, feeling and, occasionally, tasting. It is about using all our senses to understand the current environment.
- Integrating this information with relevant knowledge to create a mental picture of the current situation – identifying that all is well or identifying emerging or unexpected risks.

---

36 Dominguez, C., Vidulich, M., Vogel, E. & McMillan, G. (1994). *Situation awareness: Papers and annotated bibliography*. Armstrong Laboratory, Human System Center, ref. AL/CF-TR-1994-0085

- Using this picture to direct further perceptual exploration in a continual perceptual cycle – in other words, using all our senses and knowledge to help us monitor and have a current picture of our situation.

- Anticipating future events through those observations, and through our own and others' perceptions and knowledge, and using this to form a view of any action that might be needed or to build an ongoing awareness that all is well.

Most of us will have been on long car journeys. Many of us will have found ourselves in huge traffic delays coming down the M6 towards Birmingham. My husband and I have done it many times when travelling back from the Lake District with four young children. The driver needs situational awareness to understand the best options and to minimise risks – bored children, needing the toilet, becoming fractious. The signs of this are usually in advance of someone hitting someone else, or bursting into tears, or 'having an accident'. As parents in the front, we can react to situational signs of initial boredom with a 'Naughty Panda and Piggywig' puppet show from the passenger seat, and a promise that it won't be long until we stop. We can keep looking in the rear-view mirror and trying to see ahead. We can try and work out from previous experience whether to turn off or whether to carry on and hope it will clear.

Luckily, from 2003, we could throw the M6 Toll into our situational awareness and that allowed us to decide to stay on the motorway rather than come off. There used to be fountains outside the services that the children could play in, so they were happy with a few verses of 'Wind the Bobbin Up', a game of 'I Spy' and the times tables song tape. Actually, they were probably less excited about the times tables, but needs must. Parental situational awareness afforded us the knowledge that we had a captive audience. We could spot when our son was truly desperate as he stopped speaking, and we carried a cut-off empty lemonade bottle just in case. Getting to the services without disaster, knowing whether to stop or risk continuing, was all about situational judgement, balancing what we were experiencing and our prior knowledge.

9. Lack of knowledge

The regulatory requirements for training and qualification are significant in all types of health and social care services. Sometimes there is a crossover of responsibilities and delegation of tasks, so who can do what becomes a bit blurred. Nursing is particularly complex when considering skills mix. There are few tasks that are required to be completed by a registered nurse. There are many where one would usually expect a task to be undertaken only by someone who is a registered nurse but there are few requirements, so many providers delegate many tasks and train staff without professional regulation to carry out certain tasks. That person may be excellent at that particular task – I would much rather a hospital phlebotomist take blood (because they do it all day, every day) than a practice nurse or a newly qualified foundation-year doctor, who do it occasionally as one of their many responsibilities.

There are times when the lack of wider professional knowledge might not result in the best outcome for people using services. The wise provider looks at outcomes when deciding staffing and considers the skills mix carefully. There is evidence that adequate numbers of well-educated nurses working in acute care areas can reduce the risk of patient mortality in high-income countries.[37] This means that reducing the numbers of registered nurses and replacing them with health care assistants to decrease costs may not actually do so. Lower staffing levels of registered nurses and higher numbers of patients per registered nurse are associated with increased risk of death during an admission to hospital. There may be significant consequences of reduced nurse staffing, and research does not support policies that encourage the use of healthcare assistants to compensate for shortages of registered nurses.[38] Where there are worse outcomes, there are higher costs.

To be clear, that does not mean devaluing the role of healthcare assistants, but rather that providers and registered managers need to be considerate of the potential consequences when using unregistered nurses with less professional education than their registered colleagues.

Where staff are employed for a specific task, they may need additional training that is wider than that task to optimise outcomes for people using the service. For instance, someone employed as a kitchen assistant who always helps with lunches should have training to help them understand the safest way to assist people to eat. They should know what is expected of them if someone chokes, and understand the difference between safe food-holding temperatures and safe serving temperatures.

In a service where people may exhibit very distressed, aggressive behaviours or may self-harm, the person, the staff, and others, may be placed at risk if all staff (not just clinical staff) have not had training and competency assessment in de-escalation of violence and trigger avoidance. Here, as elsewhere, a lack of experience and specific knowledge can result in staff misjudging situations and making unsafe decisions.

It is important for employees to undertake continuing professional development and for staff to share their knowledge with each other and across the organisation. Part of this learning process should include recent

---

37   Coster S, Watkins M & Norman IJ (2018) What is the impact of professional nursing on patients' outcomes globally? An overview of research evidence. *International Journal of Nursing Studies* **78** 76-83. doi: 10.1016/j.ijnurstu.2017.10.009.

38   Griffiths P, Maruotti A, Recio A et al (2019) Nurse staffing, nursing assistants and hospital mortality: retrospective longitudinal cohort study. *BMJ Quality & Safety* **28** (8) 609-617.

incidents and the measures taken to prevent recurrence. Learning does not have to be a whole day in a classroom setting – a newsletter or manager's weekly update email (that reaches all staff) may give a summary of an incident and the action taken – for example what followed when staff assumed that someone was confused when they said they had already had their morning medication. They could discuss the incident in a staff meeting and consider ways in which the risk of recurrence could be reduced.

10. Fatigue

We all get tired sometimes and we all know that it affects our performance and can have serious consequences. A long time ago, one of our housemen was driving from London to his family home in Wales after a very busy stretch of nights, where we had fourteen children die in a week. All the deaths were unavoidable, and all were tragedies for their families. The workload for the nursing and medical staff was high, but not something that could be minimised or deferred. The houseman was exhausted; too tired to eat the toast the ward housekeeper had made for the night staff going off duty. He sat slumped, just about keeping upright in his chair during our multi-disciplinary handover. Driving home on the M4, and despite several black coffees, he felt so tired that his eyes began to close and he deemed it unsafe to continue. He pulled onto the hard shoulder somewhere near Swindon and rolled his seat back for ten minutes – a cat nap to allow him to reach the next services or junction without incident.

Unfortunately for him, the police and magistrate didn't think a gruelling week of nights was sufficient reason to stop on the hard shoulder. He escaped disqualification but was given a hefty fine and points on his licence. Usually, he was a natural conformist who kept to the rules and was a good practitioner – thoughtful, measured, knowledgeable and skilled. On this occasion, fatigue stopped him making wise decisions. He could have slept and then driven home later. He could have caught a train. He could have reacted as soon as he knew he needed a coffee to stay awake and napped at the service station. He was lucky that the only impact was to his wallet and licence. The consequences of falling asleep at the wheel could have been so much worse.

Fatigue is a normal reaction to prolonged physical or mental stress. We can become fatigued after long periods of work and also after periods of especially hard or intense work (both marathon runners and sprinters are fatigued after training sessions). As we become more fatigued, our ability to concentrate, remember and make decisions reduces. Therefore, we are more easily distracted, and we lose situational awareness.

We often underestimate our level of fatigue – who hasn't needed and found their 'second wind'? Who hasn't thought they could walk, swim or run further than they actually could? We tend to overestimate our ability to cope with fatigue, as anyone sharing a ferry across the Solent after the Isle of Wight Festival will have seen. In the work environment, it is important that managers and staff can recognise the signs and symptoms of fatigue, both in themselves and others. There is a professional responsibility to ensure that you are fit for work, and that you intervene if you have concerns about someone's fitness to practice through fatigue.

Providers and registered managers need to ensure that staff rotas and workloads do not habitually create fatigue such that it impacts on the safety of people using services. That means ensuring sufficient, suitably skilled staff. It means NHS boards listening to their Guardian of safe working hours. It means having policies about secondary employment and overtime that are enacted and monitored. It means paying particular attention to groups and tasks where the risks introduced by fatigue are particularly high – in operating theatres and other areas where interventional activities are undertaken, where staff drive, and where medicines are administered – particularly intravenous or intrathecal drugs or other fast-acting oral drugs and controlled drugs. Encouraging staff to 'sell back' their leave my seem like a benefit to both parties, but it may have untoward effects. Encouraging staff to do overtime without real limits being imposed, or not monitoring the amount of private work a surgeon or anaesthetist is undertaking, can have serious consequences.

In 2018, a thirty-four-year-old man was sent home from accident and emergency by a busy consultant. The man subsequently died from a blood clot. He had been admitted to hospital four days earlier. He was diagnosed with a blocked artery on his lung following an X-ray and had started to show signs of improvement after being treated. The patient was due to be transferred to a medical emergency assessment unit to continue his treatment, but he was discharged with antibiotics for a chest infection by an emergency department consultant. The inquest into his death heard that the doctor had had no more than two hours' sleep before he was called back into work, because there were fifty-six patients in the emergency department at the time, with sixteen more waiting to be admitted. It was concluded that the patient would have lived had he continued with the treatment for the blood clot.[39]

11. Lack of assertiveness

Being both unable to express our concerns and not allowing others to express theirs creates ineffective communication and damages teamwork. Unassertive team members can be forced to go with a majority decision, even when they believe it is wrong and dangerous to do so.

---

39   Whitelam P (2020) *Hospital patient, 34, dies three days after 'tired' doctor discharged him by mistake.* Lincolnshire Live. Available at: www.lincolnshirelive.co.uk/news/local-news/hospital-patient-34-dies-three-3867782 (accessed August 2023).

Fear of retribution has long been recognised as a reason why people working in the NHS do not speak out about concerns they may have about patient safety, as was reported in the *British Medical Journal* in 2012.[40] My own experience as a regulator has shown me that staff may be justified in being worried that if they report concerns about patient safety their career will be blighted, or their employment may become untenable. This has been the case not only in the NHS but also in independent healthcare and social care organisations. If highly qualified, competent and usually confident people are too afraid of what they may face, then how can providers expect staff who are new, less secure in their roles or financially insecure to speak out? The truth is that we often don't treat whistle-blowers very well, and sometimes we treat them very badly.

The CQC cannot afford to be complacent as there have been several well-publicised cases where the Commission has not listened when staff have raised concerns. That lack of listening results in others questioning why they should risk their careers by speaking out. It also risks missing very serious issues that result in patient harm.

My first memory of the impact of speaking up and voicing concerns was when I followed the story of the late, very courageous, Graham Pink, in the late 1980s. Graham was nursing's most famous whistle-blower. He didn't use that term and preferred 'truth-teller'. His truth was the suffering of patients due to staff shortages he witnessed when working night shifts on the elderly care wards at a Manchester hospital. He wrote letters – polite letters about the poor care – to hospital managers, civil servants and politicians, all the way up to the Prime Minister, Margaret Thatcher. He was sacked in 1991 for breaching patient confidentiality. He had never named a patient or included any confidential information in his letters.

Speaking up takes courage. We should welcome it, listen and respond. Sometimes, it is about miscommunication or misunderstanding of a rationale for changes. Sometimes it is accurate information about very real risks to safety. If staff, people using services and visitors do not feel they can voice concerns comfortably, then the provider has grown a culture that places people at increased risk. A wise provider or manager will listen. They will consider the information properly and communicate their reasoning for the actions they have taken (or the reasons why no action is necessary).

Assertiveness is a behaviour that allows us to express opinions, concerns, beliefs and needs in a productive way. It allows others to assert themselves without the recipient feeling threatened or undermined. Assertiveness is not to be confused with aggression. It is about communicating honestly and unambiguously. It is about respecting the opinions and needs of others, but not compromising our own standards.

---

40   Patrick K (2012) Barriers to whistleblowing in the NHS *BMJ* 2012; 345: e6840

Reflective practice sessions, group supervision and a strong teamworking ethos encourage people to share their thoughts and to voice concerns. As a manager, I can think of few greater compliments than one of the team phoning me to ask, "What are you thinking of?" Many is the time I have avoided mayhem and embarrassment because one of the team has given me their honest view.

12. Cultural norms – "It's just the way things are done around here"

Workplace practices develop over time. They are shaped by experience and often influenced by the workplace culture. Practice that should be consistent across a whole organisation often isn't. Sometimes, variation leads to innovation and truly personalised care, but more often inconsistent use of safety systems leads to mistakes and poor outcomes.

I can remember so many things that were described as "the way things are done around here"; most were, on reflection, and with the benefit of professional education and experience, poor practice. Some were appalling practice that I feel uncomfortable remembering. Some were good practice by guesswork and some I have never really fathomed the reason for. We used to give babies a dummy dipped in commercial rose hip syrup before and during any uncomfortable procedure. The ward sisters knew it worked from experience and learning passed down through training, but it wasn't until around 2001 that any real evidence for the use of sugar as analgesia for infants was published.[41] On the other hand, I was admitted to hospital once as a very competent and well-informed early-middle-aged woman. I was asked by the admitting student nurse how many bedrooms I had. She didn't know why she was asking, her mentor didn't know why she was asking, and the registrar doing the clerking didn't know. To this day, it seems an odd question with no purpose – it was on the form, so it was asked without any thought involved.

I also remember as a young teenager volunteering at an institution for children with learning disabilities. I was only about thirteen, but I knew there was some pretty bad care being delivered. As far as I am aware, only one of the ward sisters ever refused to follow the norms. Most staff were happy to feed the less able children a revolting mix of mashed potato, minced meat of some description, pink blancmange, and orange squash. Most were happy to hose children down rather than giving them a nice bubbly bath. Washing hair was infrequent but rough and used a grim, medicated shampoo that made the poor children scream if it got in their eyes – which it often did. After their weekly hosing, most children were given some sticky, pink liquid medicine to

---

41   Gibbins S & Stevens B (2001) Mechanisms of sucrose and non-nutritive sucking in procedural pain management in infants. *Pain Research and Management* **6** (1) 21-8. doi: 10.1155/2001/376819. PMID: 11854758.

keep them calm. It was "just the way things were done" at the home. Except by the sister who brought in her own shampoo, ran bubble baths and put music on for dancing rather than give the pink medicine. Clearly, she knew it was wrong but overcoming the "it will never work", "it's been tried before", "nobody notices" majority is hard.

Often, usual practices follow unwritten rules or behaviours, which deviate from the required rules, procedures and instructions. I inspected a large independent hospital in 2012; the norm was to not put out oxygen and suction for post-operative patients as "It made the place look like an NHS hospital." Every registered nurse knew it was wrong, but only one was brave enough to speak out and challenge "the way it is done here."

Peer pressure is powerful and can force others to go along with bad practice until it becomes habit. There will be those who will say that rules are there to be broken, but rules and procedures should be evidence-based, should comply with national guidance, and therefore ought to be enforced and followed rigorously. Where there is a 'workaround' or staff do not follow the correct procedure, the wise provider will pick this up through monitoring, communication and governance. If necessary, the procedure may need to be amended to make it easier for staff to do the right thing.

The key message is that no matter how many policies, procedures, processes, checklists and codes of practice are in place to assure safety and mitigate risk, in healthcare settings there is always one unknown factor and that is people. Safety is dependent on providers understanding human factors and ensuring that they provide a service where it is easy for people to do the right thing and avoid mistakes that have negative consequences for everyone involved. That is about recruitment, training, policies and protocols, supervision, staffing, governance and, most importantly, culture.

Chapter 8: Regulation and legislation

Sometimes it can be hard to get our heads around the language of regulation – particularly at a time of change within the regulator. As the CQC moves towards a new model of regulation, new words appear alongside those already in regular use. Different sectors have different regulatory language – core services, for example, only appear in acute healthcare settings, and the Key Lines of Enquiry (KLOEs) have been different for each sector. Those differences remain, but going forward reporting and judgement will use Quality Statements. The KLOEs are still different for each sector – a care home won't need to report 'Never Events', and an independent mobile diagnostic unit offering MRI scans won't usually need to consider nutrition and hydration.

Quality Statements are the format used to determine whether a provider is meeting the Fundamental Standards and therefore the regulations. They are the commitments that services should live up to. They are not enforceable, as they are not themselves regulations. They do not set the standards which all services should meet; they are a framework for using those standards and regulations in the inspection and monitoring processes. Quality Statements are used to determine the quality of care and treatment being provided by a service. They are the same across all provider types, although the type of assurance required may vary depending on the nature of the service. As a provider, registered manager, or leader within part of a service, you need to be able to talk about the care and treatment you provide, knowing that what you are saying is true. It is not about being perfect; no service ever is, but all services should aspire to excellence.

Celebrating success versus toxic positivity

It is a wise leader who ensures that there is current evidence demonstrating that the Quality Statements are met by their service or part of their service, and who shares this with stakeholders and regulators. Sharing good news and celebrating success is one way of building a positive culture where people feel valued. The only proviso is that shortcomings are also identified and worked on to avoid a culture of toxic positivity where raising concerns is discouraged and leadership only wants to hear and spread good news. That is very damaging, and it leads to serious failings or harms going unrecognised. It is leadership complacency at its worst; a leader who doesn't ask questions, or a board that doesn't challenge a lack of information, is not a good leader or board. If a regulator can pick up concerns about a service from nationally available data, then the board or service leaders should already be aware and responding.

A recent situation I dealt with through regulation concerned a board and system leaders who had not identified the significant under-reporting of serious incidents using the statutory NHS Serious Incident Requiring Investigation framework and database.[42] There was a culture that only told good-news stories. They were doing some very good work, and this was celebrated and circulated widely through internal means and social media. This was another service that felt it deserved an 'Outstanding' rating; there was a strong focus on innovation and being the highest performer in its service type. Staff leaders showed us some impressive data, and the board members were entirely positive about the service.

That complete lack of any risks or shortcomings led us to look closer. My husband, who has pockets of deep insight and wisdom, often says that if something looks too good to be true, it probably is. The children roll their eyes but listen and look harder. What a closer look showed us was that this provider was a significant outlier in reporting serious incidents. There are only eleven similar organisations in England, so a comparison report was quite easy to run from StEIS, the web-based serious-incident management system used by all organisations providing NHS-funded care.

Serious incidents must be reported by the provider without delay and no later than two working days after the incident is identified. Commissioners and regulators such as the CQC are able to see the information held on StEIS, although there is sometimes a time lag between reporting and appearing on the system. The Integrated Care System governance teams receive a notification of serious incidents direct from StEIS via an email to their dedicated serious-incident mailbox. If any incidents have resulted in significant harm, death or had a significant impact on service delivery, an automatic email alert is sent to the commissioners. The fail-safes in the system should mean that there is good oversight of all serious incidents that occur in services delivering care to NHS patients.

Except, of course, that human factors have an impact, and the system requires incidents to be reported in the first place. Sometimes, unless a problem is spelt out, it remains unseen and the good-news stories get traction over and above the shortcomings. This particular provider was not reporting serious incidents because they wanted to be seen to be high performing. Instead, they had created their own internal review system and renamed serious incidents as 'major' incidents (that weren't deemed reportable). This meant that their board-reporting dashboard stayed a lovely green colour, which was greeted with plaudits and no challenge.

---

42   www.england.nhs.uk/patient-safety/serious-incident-framework/ (accessed August 2023).

The real consequences, of course, were that there was no learning, no sharing of concerns and no effective internal or external governance. Thousands of safeguarding referrals were not processed due to IT system failings, but these went unreported and unactioned. Mainly because of a culture of toxic positivity where incidents were hidden rather than learned from, but also because the service's unrelenting focus on good news had 'pulled the wool over the board and commissioners' eyes' and inhibited proper challenge.

How Quality Statements link to regulations

Quality Statements are mapped to each of the five key questions ("Is it safe?"; "Is it effective?"; "Is it caring?"; "Is it responsive?"; "Is it well-led?"). There are also Quality Statements being mapped to the NHS 'well-led' part of comprehensive inspections, although that is still being tweaked. The Quality Statements sound quite simple. They are statements of one or two sentences, and it would be easy for a registered manager or provider to be complacent, read the statement and say, "Yes, we do that." The Quality Statements are how evidence is judged and reported by the Commission. Their main focus is the Fundamental Standards. In essence, the Quality Statements are the interpretation of the Fundamental Standards written into a report for publication.

Let's take the Fundamental Standard about staffing that says that care providers must only employ people who can provide care and treatment appropriate to their role. The regulation states that providers must have strong recruitment procedures in place and carry out relevant checks such as on applicants' criminal records and work history. It is easy to see that, in different settings, this needs more detail. A maternity unit cannot decide to replace midwives with paramedics. A care home may need registered nurses, but it should not use them to perform work for which they are not trained or qualified. A renal nurse may be very well-educated and a lovely person, but that doesn't make him or her suitable to employ as the clinical lead in a centre for people who have minimal consciousness or who are ventilated.

The Fundamental Standards are the standards below which care must never fall.[43] Many service leaders give a passing nod to the Fundamental Standards and think that is sufficient to get a 'Good' rating. It is, of course, entirely possible that there are sufficiently experienced staff and safety processes already established to meet the requirements of the regulation. In this situation, the human factors carry the provider because of "the way we do it around here", but there are inherent risks – not least that aiming for a 'Good' rating is indicative of complacency and increases the likelihood of falling short of that standard. Staff change over time. The needs and

---

43 www.cqc.org.uk/about-us/fundamental-standards (accessed August 2023).

expectations of service users change. Legislation changes. National guidance changes. Regulatory frameworks and inspection methodologies change. A good provider accepts that while the status quo might provide acceptable care, there are always ways to improve outcomes for people using the service, and ways to stand above the field as a centre of excellence that is recognised through regulation.

It is important to understand that the Quality Statements are not quite as simple as they sound. Each is mapped to several regulations, and it is the regulations that are enforceable. Warning notices, prosecutions, requirement notices, civil action and conditions are all pinned to the regulations rather than the Quality Statements. It is the regulations that give the authority for the CQC to act where there are care failings. They are the interpretation of the legislation, the working tools that enable compliance with the Health and Social Care Act 2008 (Regulated Activities) Regulations 2014 to be monitored and enforced. Each regulation is underpinned by guidance from the CQC. It is that guidance that inspection teams work to, and on which they base their judgements about safety and quality. The information is not secret; it is on the CQC website for all to read.[44] The page can be found by searching 'CQC Regulations'. Providers and service leaders need to understand this guidance, think how it applies to their service and ensure that they can provide evidence of compliance.

Interpreting and complying with regulations

I will not list all the regulations, as they are readily available online and providers should already be aware of them. However, it may be helpful to work through one specific regulation and think about the expectations surrounding it from a care-delivery and inspection perspective. I will use Regulation 12: 'Safe care and treatment', as this is the key regulation relating to safety. It is not the only regulation that needs to be considered with regard to the 'safe' domain, but if you follow this method of detailed consideration of CQC guidance against each regulation then you will likely find yourself providing safe care and treatment and comfortably the right side of at least a 'Good' rating. The regulation is shown in full below; the detailed CQC guidance that accompanies it can be found in the Appendix.

---

44 www.cqc.org.uk/ (accessed August 2023).

Regulation 12: Safe care and treatment

1. Care and treatment must be provided in a safe way for service users.
2. Without limiting paragraph (1), the things which a registered person must do to comply with that paragraph include—
   a. assessing the risks to the health and safety of service users of receiving the care or treatment;
   b. doing all that is reasonably practicable to mitigate any such risks;
   c. ensuring that persons providing care or treatment to service users have the qualifications, competence, skills and experience to do so safely;
   d. ensuring that the premises used by the service provider are safe to use for their intended purpose and are used in a safe way;
   e. ensuring that the equipment used by the service provider for providing care or treatment to a service user is safe for such use and is used in a safe way;
   f. where equipment or medicines are supplied by the service provider, ensuring that there are sufficient quantities of these to ensure the safety of service users and to meet their needs;
   g. (the proper and safe management of medicines;
   h. assessing the risk of, and preventing, detecting and controlling the spread of, infections, including those that are health care associated;
   i. where responsibility for the care and treatment of service users is shared with, or transferred to, other persons, working with such other persons, service users and other appropriate persons to ensure that timely care planning takes place to ensure the health, safety and welfare of the service users.

I would suggest that as a provider, registered manager or board member, or as a leader in a part of a larger organisation, you work through each regulation and its associated guidance to ensure not only that you are compliant, but also that you can evidence that you are compliant. It doesn't all have to be done at once, but it does need to be done with a willingness to identify where you may not be fully compliant or where there is scope to provide more evidence of compliance. Feed that information to the CQC via the provider portal, share it with your system leaders and commissioners, share it with staff, service users and their families or representatives. Ensure others know that you are performing well, and that you expect people to receive high-quality care and treatment. Sharing shortcomings is only a bad thing if you don't also share what you have done about it. You are unlikely to face censure for a few medication recording errors if you have investigated, identified that they all occurred on night duty when one specific person was responsible for the checks and put plans in place to reduce the risks of future errors. That might involve employing additional staff, closer supervision, a move to an automated system or retraining and competency assessment – the answer will come from the investigation. But seeing that process of governance will provide assurance, not raise the provider risk level on CQC systems.

Involve people in the development of the service and consult about how care and treatment are provided, to enable a shared view of what high-quality care looks like. Staff are far more likely to adhere to a safety system if they have been involved in its design or commissioning and understand why it is necessary. People using services are more likely to accept the need for restrictions on bath-water temperature if they understand the risk to themselves and others of unrestricted hot water temperatures.

Celebrate good news while avoiding toxic positivity – if you identify shortcomings, make sure you address them. Tell people how and when you are going to address them. Be honest: openness and transparency make for a safer, higher-quality service. If you know the water coming from the taps in your handwash basins is too hot to enable safe handwashing, tell staff how that is being addressed and when they can expect to wash their hands without risking scalds. Ensure good governance around risks and deliver plans to address shortfalls, rather than making excuses for delays. You can be sure that if you don't make improvements in a timely way, you will be required to do so through regulation and that may include enforcement.

Let's take another example of toxic positivity. A provider had a bird infestation problem in one of their ambulance stations. It was a very longstanding problem, with bizarre mitigation of risk which included staff wearing bin bags to avoid having their uniforms covered in bird droppings and teams responsible for cleaning and restocking vehicles working in respirators. Supplies were under makeshift tents and the floor was absolutely covered in droppings. The provider had known about this for a long time but, offering a variety of excuses, had failed to deal with the problem. They kept it hidden from all but those working at the station. The board didn't know about it despite there being significant risks of long-term exposure to bird droppings over and above the infection prevention and control risk. It didn't appear on any risk register.

Staff stopped reporting the concern. The provider sold a story of caring for their staff and focusing on wellbeing that was not borne out in practice. The issue was allowed to continue for years. The inevitable enforcement that followed was uncomfortable for the provider and leaders of the service, but it was also the trigger for action. Within a short time, the birds were removed. Had the leaders felt able to say that they knew about the problem, shown inspectors the discussion that had taken place through governance processes and the action taken, and offered a timeline for eradication of the birds, their report might have read a little better.

The purpose of Regulation 12 is to protect people from unsafe care and treatment. It is about reducing avoidable harm. Providers must assess the risks to people's health and safety during any care or treatment and make sure that staff have the qualifications, competence, skills and experience to keep people safe.

The guidance states that there are specific areas of risk to people's health and safety that the provider must consider and suggests that the list offered as part of Regulation 12 is not exhaustive.[45] The legal requirement is that providers must demonstrate that they have done everything reasonably practicable to provide safe care and treatment. In practice, that means that providers and registered managers really need to think about their service and the needs and preferences of the people using it. It cannot be a one-off consideration, as the needs of people change over time, as does the guidance and the law. The consideration of risk is an ongoing process, and demonstrating thar requires the management of risks at every level throughout an organisation. This probably means a risk register of some sort that shows recognition, assessment, action and review of risks both to individuals and across the organisation.

Overlap between regulations

In terms of inspection, the risk management process usually sits under Regulation 17: 'Good governance'. The risks that sit under Regulation 12: 'Safe care and treatment' are about individual risk assessments that identify each person's needs. Clearly, there is an overlap between Regulation 12: 'Safe care and treatment' and several other regulations including Regulation 9: 'Person centred care', Regulation 13: 'Safeguarding', Regulation 15: 'Premises and Equipment' and Regulation 18: 'Staffing'.

It is unlikely that people will be getting safe care in a service where there is non-compliance with other regulations. If a maternity service is habitually short-staffed, if there is no labour ward coordinator and many women do not receive one-to-one care in established labour, and if, on the postnatal and antenatal wards, there is sometimes no midwife working, then the care of women and their babies is likely suffer and outcomes may be poor, resulting in tragedies. Enforcement in this case is quite likely to be against Regulation 18: 'Staffing' rather than Regulation 12. The action that the CQC takes will be against a specific regulation, and they will usually not act against two different regulations for the same shortfall in provision.

Similarly, if a GP practice has poor governance arrangements, does not monitor outcomes for patients and is unaware that its referral rate for ovarian cancer is lower and later than that offered by most other GP services, then it is likely that women with an early ovarian cancer may be missed, and they may remain untreated until the disease is incurable. That is why good governance matters. Failure to comply with Regulation 17: 'Good governance' in this situation is also very unsafe for patients, who may not be offered the treatment they need.

---

45 Care Quality Commission (2023) *Regulation 12: Safe care and treatment* [online]. Available at: www.cqc.org.uk/guidance-providers/regulations-enforcement/regulation-12-safe-care-treatment (accessed August 2023).

If there had been good governance arrangements at Donneybrook Medical Centre in Hyde, Greater Manchester, lives would undoubtedly have been saved. This was the GP practice where Dr Harold Shipman worked. In January 2000, he was convicted of murdering fifteen of his patients by administering lethal doses of diamorphine. Further investigations estimate that, during his working life, Shipman killed about two hundred and forty of his patients, making him the most prolific serial killer in British history. In this case, the care and treatment was clearly unsafe, but the biggest provider failing was the lack of governance that allowed Shipman to continue to kill.

The regulation of Shipman's clinical practice was the responsibility of the General Medical Council. There was national learning, and following the prosecution, a public enquiry was carried out, chaired by Dame Janet Smith.[46] In response to the enquiry, the government agreed a new legislative structure to control diamorphine and other controlled drugs that have the potential to be misused. The regulations required healthcare organisations to appoint an officer to take responsibility for the safe management of controlled drugs within their organisation. The role given to the CQC was to oversee the arrangements, ensuring that the regulations were implemented.

In some cases, the Commission might use two regulations to act if there is evidence that both have been breached. That is why it is important to understand exactly which regulations are mapped to the Quality Statements, and to ensure compliance with them all. In the maternity case above, there might be action such as a Warning Notice about the lack of a labour ward coordinator and the absence of midwives on the postnatal ward against Regulation 18: 'Staffing', but a prosecution against Regulation 12: 'Safe care and treatment' where those staffing shortfalls have led to specific serious harm to a mother or baby; maybe complications were not identified by a student nurse left on their own with a birthing mother. If it is evident that after the student asked for someone to look at the monitoring records and was told that they should understand the graph at their stage in training, and after nobody answered the call bell when the student pressed it, a consequent and avoidable harm came to the baby, then a fuller investigation by the Commission and potential prosecution would be taken against Regulation 12.

Regulation and legislation

Knowing and understanding the regulations and what is required to be compliant is essential to meeting the Fundamental Standards which are so important to protecting people from avoidable harm. Providers, registered managers and leaders of areas of larger services should ensure that their knowledge remains current. They should take steps to ensure that they meet any nationally recognised guidance applicable for their service or part of a

---

46   www.cqc.org.uk/sites/default/files/20140811%20CQC%20Controlled%20drugs%20annual%20 report%202013%20final.pdf (accessed August 2023).

service. Some statutory and national guidance is applicable to all service types, and some is specific to highly specialised locations. The manager of a home for people living with dementia does not need to know the *NICE Clinical guideline [CG98]: Jaundice in new-born babies under 28 days*. The manager of a travel clinic is unlikely to need to know the details of the Human Fertilisation and Embryology Act (1990). There are, however, many areas of commonality – guidance, regulations and laws that all providers, all managers and all leaders of units within large services should at least be aware of and know where to find more information, if required.

There are also laws applicable to all service types where more than 'having heard of it' is required. Failure to properly apply the Mental Capacity Act (2005) will likely see providers face enforcement under Regulation 11: 'Consent'.[47] Failure to adhere to the safe storage of toxic and hazardous substances may be a breach of the Control of Substances Hazardous to Health Regulations (COSHH) but is also likely to be a breach of Regulation 12: 'Safe care and treatment'.[48] The list of legislation that requires compliance from providers is long and varies depending on the service type, but the key legislation that most providers must comply with to ensure they are providing a safe service that protects people from harm includes, but is not limited to:

- The Mental Capacity Act (2005)
- The Regulatory Reform (Fire Safety) Order 2005
- Control of Substances Hazardous to Health 2002
- Health and Safety at Work Act (1974)
- Manual Handling Operations Regulations 1992 (amended 2002)
- Reporting of Injuries, Diseases and Dangerous Occurrences Regulations 1995
- Health and Safety (First Aid) Regulations 1981
- Food Safety Act 1990, Food Safety (General Food Hygiene) Regulations 1995 and Food Safety (Temperature Control) Regulations 1995
- Sexual Offences Act (2003)
- Safeguarding Vulnerable Groups Act (2006) and the Protection of Freedoms Bill
- Public Interest Disclosure Act (1998)
- Human Medicines Regulations 2012

The key point with regard to the Quality Statements is that they are broad, and ensuring that a service is compliant with the Health and Social Care Act (2008) (Regulated Activities) Regulations 2014 is a complex task that requires significant

---

47 www.legislation.gov.uk/ukpga/2005/9/contents (accessed August 2023).

48 www.hse.gov.uk/coshh/basics/index.htm (accessed August 2023).

work – not only to ensure that the service meets the required standards at the point of registration, but also to ensure that it continues to do so as legislative changes are introduced. Compliance is an active and ongoing process.

Assessing and managing risks

Risk assessments relating to the health, safety and welfare of people using services must be completed and reviewed regularly by people with the qualifications, skills, competence and experience to do so. Risk assessments should include plans for managing risks. Planning and delivery of care and treatment should be based on risk assessments that balance the needs and safety of people using the service with their rights and preferences. They should also include arrangements to respond appropriately and in good time to people's changing needs in accordance with the Mental Capacity Act (2005). This includes best interest decision-making, lawful restraint, and, where required, application for authorisation for deprivation of liberty through the Mental Capacity Act (2005) Deprivation of Liberty Safeguards or the Court of Protection. All this applies when people use a service. This includes when they are admitted, discharged, transferred or move between services.

Providers must make sure that the premises and any equipment used is safe and, where applicable, available in sufficient quantities. Medicines must be supplied in sufficient quantities, managed safely and administered appropriately in order to make sure that people are safe. Providers must prevent and control the spread of infection. Where the responsibility for care and treatment is shared, care planning must be timely to maintain people's health, safety and welfare.

The CQC understands that there may be inherent risks in carrying out care and treatment, and will not consider it to be unsafe if providers can demonstrate that they have taken all reasonable steps to ensure the health and safety of people using their services and to manage risks. The Commission can prosecute for a breach of all or part of a Regulation 12: 'Safe care and treatment' if a failure to meet the regulation results in avoidable harm to a person using the service or if a person is exposed to a significant risk of harm. It does not have to serve a Warning Notice before prosecution. Additionally, the CQC may also take other regulatory action. The CQC must refuse registration if providers cannot satisfy them that they can and will continue to comply with this regulation.

Note: The regulation does not apply to the person's accommodation if this is not provided as part of their care and treatment.

Chapter 9: The Fundamental Standards – People and Places

The Fundamental Standards are, very simply, those standards below which care must never fall. They are the lower limit of acceptable care, rather than something that should be aspired to. All regulated services should meet the Fundamental Standards, all the time. In terms of importance, they are the key areas of care that providers and managers should ensure they never lose sight of, and they are the very essence of a good service. Like the Quality Statements they aren't enforceable as they are not themselves regulations, but they are the interpretation of the regulations. They state explicitly, in a very simple way, what the regulations demand of providers. If you are not meeting the Fundamental Standards, then you will be breaching at least one regulation. What level of enforcement that results in will depend on the degree of harm and risk that people using the service are exposed to.

How do the Fundamental Standards link to the new single assessment framework? That is easiest to understand if you consider that what good care looks like is reasonably well understood. There will be greater variance when we talk about outstanding practice and innovation, but everyone understands that people reliant on health and social care services should expect to have their care or treatment delivered in line with their assessed needs, for example. That applies equally to a frail elderly person relying on staff in a care home and to a child with Type 1 diabetes relying on staff to help them understand and manage their condition. The central guiding principle is the same – that needs are assessed, and care is planned.

How that is enacted and measured will vary by individual and type of service. An independent ambulance provider will not usually need to demonstrate compliance with the national guidance on laser safety, but both they and a provider of ophthalmic surgery (who does use lasers to deliver their service) will need to understand what the risks associated with their particular service type are, along with the guidance or regulations associated with that, and have some way of demonstrating that they are meeting the Fundamental Standards, that the Quality Statements apply to their service and that they are thus compliant with the regulations. There is an overlap between the Fundamental Standards and the Quality Statements, inevitably, but providers need to demonstrate they have considered both. In this chapter and the next, we will look at each of the Fundamental Standards in turn.

Person-centred care

Services should provide person-centred care and people must have care or treatment that is tailored to their needs and preferences.

This is an aspect of care that very large providers sometimes struggle with. They run on standardised processes and pathways and there can sometimes be resistance to personalising the care they provide; indeed, it is often argued that standardisation promotes safety in complex treatment delivery. That is a misunderstanding of the notion of personalised care and what is a reasonable expectation.

Yet it is not just the big providers that have problems. Many, many providers fall short on this, and luckily for them, it often isn't reported on. Health inequalities comes to mind. There are several key safety considerations that are needed in order to ensure safe and equitable care, but we are only just beginning to see these inequalities being addressed. Does your pressure damage prevention policy and training identify the appearance of damage to different coloured skin? Similarly, while there have been significant improvements in the way services meet the needs of people with learning disabilities or autism, there is still a long way to go.

A good while ago, when inspecting a children's unit at a district general hospital, a mother told me that she was exhausted and exasperated as she could not leave her fourteen-year-old autistic son alone on the ward while she went to the lavatory, made a cup of tea, or had a meal in peace. He had a mattress on the floor, as he was unable to use an ordinary hospital bed and there was no special high-sided bed available for him. This meant that if she left his side, he wandered off and put himself at risk of harm. Twice in the week, she took him home for a bath as there was no suitable bathroom for him on the unit. There was no changing table or space in the bathroom, and so she changed him bending down over the mattress on the floor. She described the staff as lovely and caring, and the hospital as brilliant. She felt like one of the family on the ward, but her back was hurting and she was close to tears with tiredness.

I invited the Chief Nurse to come and have a mug of tea with me and the mother – a far more effective strategy than a requirement notice in a report. She immediately understood that this six-foot tall, fourteen-stone child needed something more than a dinosaur counterpane. She spoke with a local children's hospice where the lad sometimes had respite care and arranged for him to be transferred there, because they had more appropriate equipment and facilities. They agreed to offer acute care as a short-term measure after talking to me about the impact and regulatory requirements, and the on-call paediatrician agreed to do an off-site ward round. Longer term, the hospital's children's team worked with the hospice and the parent to ensure that they identified the most appropriate equipment and resources to enable the hospital to meet the needs of older children with complex needs.

Improved safety through personalised care needs providers and staff to stop, think and listen to people to ensure they really are thinking about the people using the service. Why do children routinely get a parent to accompany them to theatre, but a confused and frightened elderly person can't have their spouse or adult daughter? Some places say they will allow it, if asked, but why do we wait until people find the courage to ask? Why are staff not offering this routinely? It would be kinder for sure, but it would also be safer for all involved. The accompanying adult might well reduce agitation by their presence, and so reduce the risk of assaults on staff, allegations of harm or people hurting themselves on trolley rails or by falling. If there is someone accompanying the person who knows them well, then 'Never Events' around wrong site surgery might be less of a risk because the accompanying person will be able to say, through the heightened tension created by a very distressed person, that it is actually the left eye being treated not the right. If a GP surgery uses a professional interpreter, rather than relying on a spouse, they might reach an accurate diagnosis more easily and not be fobbed off by an anxious partner whose anxiety management strategy is to minimise.

There are many examples of excellence in ensuring personalised care. They aren't always recorded or shared with inspections teams, so others don't see the possibilities and there is limited shared learning. Such a waste of excellence!

On an engagement visit to Conquest Hospital in Hastings, which at the time faced its own challenges, I met a young man with autism and his parents. They were about to leave after surgery and wanted to stop off and say thank you to the Chief Nurse who had persuaded teams to work together to enable the young man to have the surgery he needed. I can't recall the type of surgery, but I can remember that the anaesthetist and an operating department assistant had seen the young man for a pre-operative assessment in the hospital car park. The Trust had arranged for this rather than him having to attend on a different day for the assessment. No gowns were required, no sitting around on the day surgery unit waiting to be called, nothing that frightened him or triggered distressed behaviour. His mother had weighed him at home, and this was accepted as sufficiently accurate. Both parents walked him into the anaesthetic room and, despite him being nineteen years old, the room was filled with things he liked, and which made him feel safe. He was put under wearing his jogging trousers and a zipped-up hoody. They could be removed quickly enough after he was anaesthetised. Gas was used to send him off before a cannula was inserted and bloods taken.

Every person involved really thought about what was right for this young man. He still followed the same care pathway, but some extra precautions were taken that acknowledged his autism and the risks it posed if he had not received personalised care. He may well not have gone through with surgery, or he might have become very distressed and potentially violent.

Personalised care really is safer care.

Dignity and respect

People must be treated with dignity and respect at all times while receiving care and treatment. This includes making sure people have privacy when they need and want it, and ensuring everybody is treated as equals. People should be given any support they need to help them remain independent and involved in their local community.

This doesn't sound much like risk reduction and safety at first glance, does it? I don't think I have ever met a health or social care professional who doesn't think they offer this. Sadly, that is not the case, and I have seen more flesh and witnessed personal distress far more often than I should have. We know it is the right thing to do but we still don't do it, possibly because we stop seeing the person and focus on the task.

Should an elderly woman with advanced dementia, being cared for at the end of her life, be strip-washed with the door open by a male carer because she won't know? Should an elderly man be encouraged to use a commode beside a bed because it is easier than supporting him to walk to the lavatory? How private are the consulting rooms in your GP practice? Are there locks and curtains to protect the privacy of patients being seen by the practice nurse?

How can these be safety risks? If you stop, reflect and ask yourself what the person's reaction would be, the risks become clearer. Imagine a recently married Muslim or Brethren woman attending for her first cervical smear. If she isn't comfortable because the doors don't lock, and she feels exposed because a curtain isn't pulled around the examination couch, she might well think that her risk is so low as to be negligible and not return. And of course she might be right, unless her husband has transmitted the HPV virus from a previous sexual encounter. Her risk increases, and, if she doesn't accept screening because of a perceived lack of privacy, then she isn't receiving safe care and treatment, is she?

Similarly, if a GP is rushed and isn't allowing their patient whose first language is not English to take their time to interpret and explain their symptoms properly, a minor heart attack might be dismissed as indigestion. It is not beyond the realms of possibility to think that the same patient may arrive too late at an emergency department to be offered life-saving treatment a few weeks later.

Even ignoring someone's preferred name presents safety risks (as well as being just plain rude). The perceived norm nowadays is that everyone wants to be called by their first name, and very rarely are people actually asked what their preference is. Calling Dr Groves by his first name, Edward, when he has never been called Edward in his entire 68-year-long life may mean he is confused when something is asked of him. Had he been called Dr Grove or even Ted, he might have been able to respond. He might not have become distressed because the tablets the nurse was trying to give him were for some chap called Edward and he was worried that they were making a serious mistake. He might not have lashed out to protect himself, putting himself and the staff member at risk. All because they didn't bother to check his preferred name.

I've only come across one care home where the matron was insistent that, unless the service user specifically asked a named member of staff to use their first name (or another less-formal name), that they were addressed by their title and surname. Most people living in the home were really pleased to be shown the respect they felt that showed, and most chose to continue to be addressed formally.

Failing to protect the privacy and dignity of people is a failure to identify consequent risk, and to provide safe care and treatment.

Consent

Provider and staff must ensure that people give consent before any care or treatment.

Most providers have systems to ensure that people give consent prior to any care or treatment. Similarly, most health and social care professionals have a good understanding of their professional codes of practice and do seek informed consent from the people they are working with. However, there are still pockets where the complexity of consent legislation and guidance makes it more challenging for staff to ensure they have been given informed consent. Are there associated safety implications? Of course there are.

There are two particularly challenging areas concerning consent. The first concerns teenagers with mental health problems in acute settings, where staff have to try and get their heads around the Mental Health Act (1983) and the law on detention, balanced against the requirements of the Mental

Capacity Act (2005) and the guidance on Gillick Competence, along with an understanding that parental responsibility includes the right of parents to consent to treatment on behalf of their children, provided the treatment is in the interests of the child.[49, 50] Each case will be different, and each person involved will likely have a different view. It's an increasing problem as more children are detained on the children's wards of acute hospitals because of a lack of mental health beds. If staff are not completely comfortable with the framework, there is a risk that a teenager will be assumed to be competent to consent and allowed to leave the ward. Perhaps worse still, older children are often placed on adult wards when they reach sixteen years of age, where there are significant safety risks because of the reduced security and oversight.

The other particularly challenging area – probably more common, but less discussed – is around the idea of 'next-of-kin'. Staff sometimes conflate someone claiming they are the next-of-kin with someone having a registered Lasting Power of Attorney for health and welfare. Some providers check the documents, but many do not, and this can lead to decisions being made that are not in the person's best interest and which are not necessarily safe. Of course, staff should be consulting with family members and other significant people who can help them understand what the person they are treating or caring for would want, if they had capacity; the problem occurs when family members disagree as to what is best, or when they are considering their own best interests and not those of the person who they claim to represent. This might take the form of financial abuse and siphoning off money for personal use as they have access to the person's account and debit card. It might be trying to avoid payment for care and treatment that the person needs, or it might be an inability to come to terms with the loss of a parent or partner, so they apply pressure for inappropriate treatment and artificially extend the person's life in a way that robs that person of dignity and a peaceful death.

Safety

Staff must not give unsafe care or treatment nor put people at risk of harm that could be avoided. Providers must assess the risks to your health and safety during any care or treatment and make sure their staff have the qualifications, competence, skills and experience to keep you safe.

This one feels very obvious in the context of a book about recognising and reducing risks. I won't labour the point.

49 NHS (2022) *Mental Health Act* [online]. Available at: www.nhs.uk/mental-health/social-care-and-your-rights/mental-health-and-the-law/mental-health-act/ (accessed August 2023).

50 NHS (2022) *Children and young people: Consent to treatment* [online]. Available at: www.nhs.uk/conditions/consent-to-treatment/children/ (accessed August 2023).

Safeguarding from abuse

People using services must not suffer any form of abuse or improper treatment while receiving care. This includes neglect, degrading treatment, unnecessary or disproportionate restraint, and inappropriate limits on people's freedom.

Only the very worst providers would not meet this standard; there is nothing you have to think about, surely? Of course, all inspections of all service types will want to know that you have appropriate safeguarding arrangements to ensure that people are protected. This means more than a piece of paper showing the dates that the three staff members completed some online training. It needs to be a full cycle of safeguarding governance, and all staff need to understand their role in protecting people. There needs to be a clear and current policy that aligns with the national guidance and appropriate training, for sure. In order to go the extra mile, there needs to be wider consideration of what this Fundamental Standard means and how providers and managers can ensure they are meeting it.

Unnecessary restraint is not just about people being pinned in a headlock or forced to the floor by four burly chaps. It's not likely to be a problem in a travel clinic or a dermatology clinic, but in a residential care home, community hospital or acute hospital – possibly. It used to be heavy, plastic-coated chairs which could be tipped back to a semi-reclining position. People were pinned in with seat belts so they couldn't get up or wander around. Dreadful for pressure damage, but that isn't the point here. So what happens now to stop people moving around and, theoretically, make life easier for staff? Bed rails used when not necessary to discourage people from leaving their bed. Staff 'tidying' walking aids so they are out of reach. Seating that is so low that people cannot get up without assistance. Lifts that require a key to be operated and which limit people from going out for a walk without 'permission'. A lovely garden made inaccessible to the majority because steps were built instead of a ramp or because doors need a code to be opened. All very common practice, and all imposing restrictions on people's liberty unless appropriate processes have been followed to protect people who lack the capacity to make the decision safely.

When we think of degrading treatment, we might well think of Winterbourne View or Whorlton Hall.[51, 52] Indeed, they were horrific

---

51   Gov.uk (2012) *Winterbourne View Hospital: Department of Health review and response* [online]. Available at: www.gov.uk/government/publications/winterbourne-view-hospital-department-of-health-review-and-response (accessed August 2023).

52   www.cqc.org.uk/news/stories/cqc-publishes-independent-review-its-regulation-whorlton-hall-between-2015-2019

examples of degrading treatment to particularly vulnerable groups. All providers need to ensure that they have ways of being certain that the people using their service are not subject to degrading treatment. They need to protect people from the development of closed cultures and make sure that staff are supported, and that the organisation is led in such a way that people remain at the core of service delivery – that they are seen as individuals and not chores to be got through. "Number 16 needs feeding" or "Bed 7 has soaked the bed again" is not a way any member of staff should talk about people using their service.

Degrading treatment can creep in when staff are working under such pressure that they stop seeing the people; when their vulnerabilities have become another inconvenience and their support needs are just a chore to be got through. One of the best examples of preventing degrading treatment was at East Surrey Hospital in Redhill. They encouraged all staff to be involved in quality improvement and to offer their ideas and suggestions. One health care assistant was concerned at the length of time it took to assemble all the essentials to provide care for someone who had suffered an episode of diarrhoea and soiled the bed or trolley. Each thing needed was in a different place. It took a while to collect them all, and meanwhile the patient was sat in a mess, distressed, uncomfortable and at increased risk of skin breakdown.

Their very simple offering was a 'diarrhoea pack' where all the required items were packed together and stored centrally so that staff could just grab a pack and begin making the patient more comfortable in a timelier way. It saved a lot of time, allowed a more relaxed approach to supporting the patient, relieved the staff frustration of not being able to find things, reduced skin breakdown and was generally better for everyone – not least the patients, whose embarrassment was relieved far more quickly. It's not degrading to have 'had an accident', but it is most certainly degrading to be left sitting in a malodorous mess for longer than is essential. Leaving someone so long that their bedding has dried after an accident is neglect, and all the policies and brightly coloured training matrices in the world don't change that. Increasingly, inspection teams will be reporting on observed care and outcomes, meaning that the quality and safety of a service will not be judged by the availability of documents.

Food and drink

Providers must ensure that people have enough to eat and drink to keep them in good health while they receive care and treatment.

Malnutrition, with and without associated disease, is a common clinical, public health and economic problem, with an estimated cost of £19.6 billion in England in 2011-12.[53]

On the whole, adult social care services and hospices are well ahead of acute hospitals when it comes to meeting this Fundamental Standard. It is not simply about offering a menu with choices that meet the needs of vegetarians, people wanting Kosher or Halal food, people who are coeliac or gluten intolerant and people who require soft diets. That is all essential, obviously (although if you know that none of your fifteen residents would choose Kosher food, then you do not need to provide it – it's not about offering everything, but about meeting the needs and preferences of people using the service). If you do have people who want a Kosher diet, then you might need to follow the full rules of kashrut. That might mean not cooking or serving dairy and meat products together.

In terms of safety, does it make a difference? If someone is not served food they can eat then, yes, it is a safety issue. To put it in context, in 2017, more than nine hundred hospital inpatients had malnourishment, dehydration or choking mentioned as a main or contributing factor on their death certificates. Of these, there were seventy-four cases where lack of food was the primary cause.[54] Some of those patients undoubtedly had complex nutritional needs and underlying morbidity that increased their risk of malnutrition, but it's still an uncomfortable statistic.

People reliant on domiciliary care services are also at increased risk of malnutrition and dehydration, not because the agencies are providing a poor service, but because people are left for extended periods without being able to access nutritious and appealing food and drink easily. A ready-meal of trout fillet in a lemon sauce, served with mashed potato, broccoli, green beans and peas warmed through in the microwave and left for the person to eat after the carers have helped them to the lavatory and given them their medicines might sound nice. Congealed and soggy mashed potato with a tiny bit of fish and mushy vegetables are not necessarily going to be wolfed down though. Even if the plate is scraped clean, it only offers 349 calories. Malnutrition is almost guaranteed.

53　Bapen (2016) *The cost of malnutrition in England and potential cost savings from nutritional interventions* [online]. Available at: www.bapen.org.uk/resources-and-education/publications-and-reports/malnutrition/cost-of-malnutrition-in-england (accessed August 2023).

54　BSNA (2019) *Report on malnutrition in NHS hospitals* [online]. Available at: https://bsna.co.uk/news/2019/report-on-malnutrition-in-nhs-hospitals (accessed August 2023).

With poor food provision and inadequate consideration of hydration comes an increased risk of all manner of ills. Pressure damage, low blood pressure and consequent dizziness and falls, urinary tract infections and acute kidney injury are but a few.

If people are not supported and assisted to eat and drink, then there are immediate risks over and above the risks of malnutrition and dehydration. If liquid-food serving temperatures are too hot, people are at risk of scalding. If swallowing assessments are not completed and the advice of speech and language therapists is not followed, people are at risk of choking. If food is not stored properly, then there is an increased risk of illnesses from pathogens. In 2019, six people died after eating pre-packed sandwiches and salads linked to a listeria outbreak at several UK hospitals. There was no suggestion of failings by the Trusts, but all hospitals used the same supplier.

In 2019, one hundred and eighty individuals aged over sixty-five years died from choking in hospital. A hospital setting is the most likely place to die of choking – it happens in hospital more than anywhere else, including at home. Care homes are also a risk, with sixty deaths occurring in the same year due to choking on food or other small objects.[55]

Food is most definitely a safety issue.

Premises and equipment

Providers must ensure that places where people receive care and treatment and the equipment used in it must be clean, suitable, and looked after properly. The equipment used to provide care and treatment must also be secure and used properly.

Clearly, this is a real safety issue, and it is important to understand that the CQC is not the sole regulator when it comes to premises and equipment safety. The need to ensure that equipment is provided and maintained to ensure that people and staff are safe should be a given, but sadly that is not always the case.

In 2019, a company was convicted of corporate manslaughter after a vulnerable elderly woman suffered burns while being bathed. An elderly resident who had advanced dementia and was losing the ability to communicate was bathed by two carers who failed to properly check the water temperature and continued to add hot water. She sustained burns across twelve percent of her body and died in hospital three days later. The

---

55   CE Safety (2019) *Report: The Un-Usual Suspects – main causes of choking deaths in the UK* [online]. Available at https://cesafety.co.uk/news/choking-deaths-report/ (accessed August 2023).

provider pleaded guilty to corporate manslaughter and was fined £1.04 million. The care home manager admitted failing to discharge a duty to take reasonable care for the health and safety of a resident and was sentenced to nine months in prison, suspended for eighteen months. A member of the care staff also admitted failing to take reasonable care for the health and safety of the resident and was sentenced to sixteen weeks in prison, suspended for eighteen months.

All for want of a water thermometer and proper monitoring that it was being used. Daily checks and the governance of such basics can be seen as tedious, and not a priority, until things go wrong. I rather imagine that with hindsight the manager wished they had insisted on seeing that bath temperature checks were completed and recorded each week. I hope the provider also wishes that they had ensured a thermostatically controlled mixer tap; it would have been much cheaper than the fine. Safe care costs less.

There needs to be a system established that allows easy oversight of the availability and safety of all the essential equipment and the premises. That way, any problems are quickly identified and addressed. People receive safe care. Staff are supported to provide that safe care and are happier in their work and there is less risk of negligence claims. The NHS paid £2.4 billion in clinical negligence claims in 2018-19, according to NHS Resolution (formerly the NHS Litigation Authority).[56]

It's not just people using the service who get compensation for their injuries. In 2019, a staff nurse who was left with chronic pain after a chair collapsed under him at work was awarded damages and costs of half a million pounds. The nurse was working a night shift in 2013 when he sat down for a rest on a 'defective' chair, which collapsed and tipped him onto the floor. He sustained what at first appeared to be a relatively minor back injury, but subsequently developed chronic pain syndrome, which meant that he was unable to work and needed to use a wheeled walking frame.

Providers and service leaders need to ensure that they are compliant with all the legislation relating to the safety of the environment and equipment. While the CQC may not be the lead regulator for some aspects of environmental safety, inspection teams have memorandums of understanding with many other agencies and will share information when they identify problems. That might be seeing damaged intumescent strips in fire-safety doors, or it might be poor food hygiene. Sometimes, providers and managers don't see themselves as responsible for things that are not within their immediate span of responsibilities – but they are. In the case of the sandwiches causing listeria deaths, the food-hygiene problems sat

---

56 Gov.uk (2019) *Annual Reports and Accounts: 2018/19* [online]. Available at: https://assets. publishing.service.gov.uk/government/uploads/system/uploads/attachment_data/file/824345/ NHS_Resolution_Annual_Report_and_accounts_print.pdf (accessed August 2023).

with the third party who provided them, but the NHS Trust staff who served them were responsible for ensuring that they reacted appropriately when it became apparent there was a problem (as they did). They also had responsibilities for the governance of food safety and oversight of the contractual arrangements.

If equipment is leased (such as a laser for use in ophthalmic surgery), the independent hospital provider using the equipment cannot simply abdicate all responsibility to the company hiring it to them. They retain a responsibility for the safe use of the equipment while it is on their premises and being used on their patients. The leasing company can offer support, training, maintenance and expert advice, but responsibility for safety ultimately remains with the hospital.

All providers and registered managers need to make sure that they have a system for ensuring they meet the requirements for fire safety, environmental health (including food safety), water safety, electrical and gas safety, medicines safety, lifting and moving equipment safety, safety relating to specialist equipment such as lasers, pressure-relieving mattresses, beds, wheelchairs, lifts, gardening machinery and laundry machinery, and safety relating to just about everything else going on in their service. Much of that will be offered by third parties – the fire-safety-equipment checks will be tested and logged by a fire-safety company, for example – but the responsibility remains with the provider to ensure that the third-party company is adhering to the contract and making the necessary checks.

An independent ambulance provider cannot blame a garage for worn tyres unless the garage has been contracted to check them weekly and this is recorded as having been done. A care home cannot blame a community Trust for supplying an alternating air-pressure-relieving mattress with a faulty motor if they still put it under someone at heightened risk who developed significant pressure damage.

The responsibility remains with the provider.

Chapter 10: The Fundamental Standards – Practices and Procedures

The previous chapter looked at the first seven Fundamental Standards – those relating to how providers make provision for, approach and treat the people who use their services. There are six further Fundamental Standards, which will be considered in this chapter – they relate to the long-term processes that providers must have in place with regard to areas like complaints, governance, recruitment and transparency.

Complaints

People must be able to complain about their care and treatment. Providers must have a system in place to handle and respond to complaints. They must investigate it thoroughly and act if problems are identified.

Too often providers, managers and staff become defensive if someone raises a concern. They say the right words to the inspection teams asking about openness and transparency, but then are abrupt or truly dismissive of anyone complaining. That is superficially understandable as nobody likes criticism; we are all prone to be defensive about our work. However, it is also a bit myopic and doesn't help to build a learning culture. Is it a safety issue, though? I am certain it is, and a poor reaction to complaints tends to make me dig a little deeper into how well the service responds to serious incidents, to allegations against staff (from service users or other staff) and to risks.

As I write this book, police are reviewing the deaths of hundreds of patients at a community hospital in Hampshire and say they have identified nineteen suspects. An independent investigation was launched into Gosport War Memorial Hospital after inquiries found that hundreds of patients had their lives shortened through the use of opioid drugs. The report of the Independent Panel says that they concluded that the lives of over four hundred and fifty patients were shortened while in the hospital. Later in the summary, the Right Reverend James Jones, the panel chair, says:

"There was a disregard for human life and a culture of shortening the lives of a large number of patients by prescribing and administering 'dangerous doses' of a hazardous combination of medication not clinically indicated or justified. They show too that, whereas a large number of patients and their relatives understood that their admission to the hospital was for either rehabilitation or respite care, they were, in effect, put on a terminal care pathway."

The documents reviewed by the panel showed that, when relatives complained about the safety of patients and the appropriateness of their care, they were consistently let down by those who should have listened and acted. Those who failed patients and their families included the senior management of the hospital, healthcare organisations, Hampshire Constabulary, local politicians, the coronial system, the Crown Prosecution Service, the General Medical Council and the Nursing and Midwifery Council. The report says that all of the individuals and agencies failed to act in ways that would have better protected patients and relatives, whose interests some subordinated to the reputation of the hospital and the professions involved.[57]

The irony is, of course, that far from protecting their reputation, they caused untold damage, allowed more patients to die before their time, and lost credibility and trust because they failed to respond appropriately to complaints. Avoidable death is obviously a safety issue and one that can sometimes be mitigated (or, at least, recurrence can be prevented) by listening and responding to people voicing concerns.

The reports of most national inquiries into health and social care scandals contain details of individuals and organisations not listening, ignoring people who raise concerns and trying to avoid the truth that is in plain sight to protect the organisational reputation. Sadly, that refusal to engage openly, to hear and consider the concerns properly, does anything but protect reputations. We have all, I am sure, heard of 'Mid-Staffs' and tend to think 'not on my watch'. Sadly, it was on some people's watch and some of those individuals and organisations tried to shut down anyone who complained. A new group, 'Cure the NHS', was formed in 2007 in the aftermath of the death of founder Julie Bailey's mother following an eight-week stay at Stafford Hospital.

Julie's tale is exceptionally sad and details the degrading, unkind and neglectful treatment her mother experienced before her death. It also shows the damage that dismissing complaints can cause. During the first few days following their mother's admission, the family came to realise that the care was unsafe; subsequent reports revealed that there were no safety systems used in some areas of the hospital. The family were so concerned about the appalling care and the way other patients were being treated they refused to leave their mother's side. Julie and her family remained in the hospital for their mother's entire stay. They were horrified at what they saw.

Following her mother's death, Julie contacted the then-CEO Martin Yeates, telling him that the hospital was a dangerous place, but received no response. She also spoke to the Director of Nursing, Helen Moss, and the local Labour MP, David Kidney. Both dismissed her concerns. Not giving up, she contacted

57 Gosport Independent Panel (2018) *The Panel Report – 20th June 2018* [online]. Available at: www.gosportpanel.independent.gov.uk/panel-report/foreword-section/foreword/ (accessed August 2023).

the local authority's Overview and Scrutiny Committee made up of Stafford borough councillors – she received a solicitor's letter back, warning her not to contact them again. All of these people and organisations failed patients, causing irreparable harm to them and also to themselves. In fact, the organisation's reputation was so damaged by the reports and inquiry's findings that it no longer exists; Stafford Hospital is now called County Hospital and is part of University Hospitals of North Midland NHS Trust.

Not addressing complaints properly, a defensive attitude, and unwillingness to hear problems causes avoidable harm and does nothing to protect individual or organisational reputations.

Good governance

Providers of care must have effective governance and systems to check on the quality and safety of care. These must help the service improve and reduce any risks to your health, safety and welfare.

This is often an area in which providers, large and small, find they are facing enforcement action. There are differences between the way a large provider needs to demonstrate that they are meeting this standard and the way a smaller provider might provide evidence that they meet it. There are also differences in the way the Commission identifies shortcomings. A large NHS Trust or corporate provider of social care will have very complex governance systems, some statutory and some for their own benchmarking or required for contractual assurance by the Integrated Care Systems (ICS). The issue for these providers is the provider (the board or the company) knowing that the information they are receiving is an accurate reflection of the service quality they are delivering. Often, staff lower down the organisational hierarchy don't escalate risk appropriately and the provider is agog when the Commission staff point out risks that they should have known about.

The reasons for not escalating 'bad news' are complex, but all result from a disconnect between board and front-line operational staff. Sometimes, it is ambitious middle managers not wanting to be seen to have problems on their watch; sometimes staff stop reporting things because they feel nothing gets done or they have seen others who raise concerns suffer detrimental treatment. Sometimes, it is a case of toxic positivity – executive staff only accepting good-news stories and trying to present an entirely positive impression of their organisation, so staff stop telling them their concerns. Good news is good, but only if it isn't used to hide safety shortcomings. A culture where staff trust their leaders, where leaders are visible and approachable, and where staff are encouraged to offer a view is likely to be a safer culture.

Smaller providers may find that governance is something they haven't really done much of previously. They may not have the scale of service or financial resources to invest in complex IT systems that allow monitoring of every time someone enters the medicines room or to run a call-bell response time report. Yet they still need to demonstrate that they are monitoring the quality and safety of care, and that they are using that monitoring to improve the care and treatment people receive.

Usually, a provider with two ambulances (that they operate themselves with just four other part-time staff members) will know that they need to comply with the statutory requirements around vehicle safety and maintenance, and around procurement and use of medicines. They often fall down on other aspects of governance, as much of what they do is done through verbal communication and taking immediate action to address things. An inspection team may be told that the service doesn't get many complaints and deals with anything straight away, that the staff are happy, and that the patients give very good feedback. The problem will be that there are no records to support that claim. If there are no complaint records (or a book which shows that there haven't been any complaints) then there is no actual evidence or ability to corroborate what the provider says.

It isn't difficult to get a hardbound book with numbered pages that can be used for any complaints to be logged and a record of action taken and outcomes to be recorded. If there are no complaints, then a simple monthly entry of date and 'No complaints received' shows that the provider understands the need to consider complaints. If there is a leaflet that can be given to people who complain that explains the complaints process, how it will be dealt with and timescales, so much the better. Governance doesn't need to be complex for smaller providers, but it does need to be evidenced. A provider that can hand over a book and say that they have not had any complaints for sixteen months – and that the complaint then was about delays to a journey which, when investigated, was shown to be caused by local roadworks – is going to get a better report than someone that says, "We don't get many complaints – in fact I can't remember the last one."

Unless there are effective governance arrangements, the service is unlikely to be safe. Certainly, the provider cannot demonstrate it is safe. The best providers not only understand their own service, but also understand how they are performing against similar services and understand any variations. Larger providers have many easier ways of benchmarking, by comparing different services under the same ownership or by comparing different units within the same service. That might be a system to identify and understand why one of a Trust's hospitals has had three 'Never Events' in a six-month period and the other two hospitals haven't, or why one care home has reported five grade-three pressure wounds when other care homes in the group have not reported any.

Governance and the good use of data to gain assurance is about asking questions. Sometimes board reports will show a number on a dashboard as assurance – it might even show numbers over several months, but often there is no real context to that. Providers and directors need to ask questions. A recent example is an Integrated Care System that failed to recognise that a Trust was an outlier for their reporting of serious incidents. The board saw very low levels of reporting as a good thing, and had set a RAG-rated target to try and show that reporting serious incidents above a certain level was a bad thing. Nobody on the board or within the system had asked the very obvious question as to where they sat in relation to others. Everyone has accepted the narrative that low reporting was an accurate reflection of the care and treatment provided. The comparative data was readily available from the national reporting system, but nobody had looked at it.

This Trust was reporting about a quarter of the number of serious incidents that similar Trusts were reporting, yet nobody asked how or why. If the service really had been that good, then others could perhaps have improved the way they worked through sharing of learning, but that wasn't the case. They weren't identifying and reporting incidents in line with the national framework. Serious incidents were being disguised by being taken outside of the correct process and only considered within the organisation. They weren't reporting these to the board, who remained unaware until it was pointed out to them. The safety risk is that very serious matters, such as failed defibrillators, were not being investigated and addressed. These governance failings were putting lives at risk, solely in order to protect an organisation's reputation.

Staffing

Providers must ensure that they have enough suitably qualified, competent, and experienced staff to make sure they can meet the Fundamental Standards. Their staff must be given the support, training and supervision they need to help them do their job.

This seems obvious, but in practice it is increasingly complex. More and more providers of health and social care services are using staff in different ways to try and meet the needs of people using their services. It's not so long ago that if you went to your GP practice, you saw a GP unless you'd made an appointment with a nurse. Now we don't have enough GPs (in April 2023 we had the equivalent of 2,133 fewer fully qualified, full-time GPs compared to the September 2015 baseline), and so the staffing model has had to change.[58] While the GP workforce is declining, the number of patients continues to rise. In April 2023, a record-high of over 62.4 million patients were registered

---

58 BMA (2023) *Pressures in general practice data analysis* [online]. Available at: www.bma.org. uk/advice-and-support/nhs-delivery-and-workforce/pressures/pressures-in-general-practice-data-analysis (accessed August 2023).

in England. As a result, the average number of patients that each full-time equivalent GP is responsible for continues to rise, and currently stands at 2,292, an increase of 355 patients per GP, or 18.3%, since 2015.

GPs can only spread themselves so far, and today we must accept that we will not always see our own GP when we want. Nurses, paramedics, pharmacists, dieticians, physiotherapists and physician's associates are all being employed in general practice to relieve the burden on doctors, and to provide advice and treatment. Usually, these are well qualified and very capable practitioners with specific expertise that they use for the benefit of patients. A pharmacist may well be better placed to complete a review of someone's complex medication to try and minimise side effects and interactions. A practice nurse with a specific interest in the care of people living with dementia may be very well placed to set up and signpost people to all the available support when a family member is first diagnosed.

Sometimes, though, a doctor's greater knowledge of the weird and wonderful is needed, and there is a risk that serious illness can be missed, or correct referral and treatment deferred for longer than if a qualified GP had seen a person sooner. Physician associates, for example, train over two years while a GP trains for a minimum of ten years, often longer. While the associate can undoubtedly support GPs, they cannot replace them as they do not have the same depth and breadth of underpinning knowledge and experience. It is for the GP partners and providers to ensure that they maintain safe staffing levels, not only in terms of numbers but in terms of how they are deployed to ensure the best outcomes for people using services.

Similarly, many tasks that once fell to registered nurses in hospitals are now carried out by healthcare assistants. Undoubtedly, healthcare assistants have a very valuable role to play, but providers cannot simply replace registered nurses without impacting on patient outcomes. Higher registered-nurse staffing levels are associated with lower avoidable mortality. Increasing registered nursing staff by an hour for each patient per day could reduce the risk of death by 3%. Increases in nursing skill mix, by having proportionately more registered nurses, may also be cost-effective. Over time, we have come to accept lower patient to nurse ratios, despite a high ratio of patients to nurses in hospitals contributing to poor patient care and increased patient mortality. The number of acute admissions has increased by 21% over the past decade, while the number of nurses caring for adults in hospitals increased by just 8%.

A study by the National Institute for Health and Care Research (NIHR) showed that:[59]

- For each day that the staffing level of registered nurses was below the average for that ward, the risk of death during the first five days of admission increased by 3%. Similarly, the risk increased by 4% for each day that the healthcare assistant staffing level was below average.

- Each additional hour worked by registered nurses per patient each day reduced the risk of death by 3%. A higher number of hours worked by registered nurses per patient each day was associated with fewer missed observations in sicker patients. No effect on risk of death was seen for additional healthcare assistant hours worked per patient each day.

The statistical model used by NIHR suggested that if there were a 0.32 increase in registered nurse staffing levels and a similar decrease in healthcare assistants (so that the skill-mix was in line with that planned by the Trust), this could reduce the death rate by 2%. It could avoid fifty deaths per year and prevent 4,464 bed-days. Though staff costs would increase by £28 per patient, overall costs would decrease due to the much lower number of bed-days. A compelling argument for not reducing registered nurse staffing as part of efficiency-saving measures!

Providers need to show that they are employing enough staff, and to do this they must show they have planned the number of staff required and can adapt staffing levels if the needs of the service or patients change. If a care home has several people who develop distressed behaviour that could result in harm to others, they are likely to need a higher staff ratio to allow for more one-to-one care, or to provide distraction to de-escalate violent behaviours. If the area serviced by a semi-rural GP practice has a new estate built with 1,200 new homes, they may need to plan how they will ensure they have sufficient resources to manage the increase in patient numbers.

Safe staffing is one area of service provision where scrimping is likely to see increased costs rather than greater efficiency. Low staff levels see more complaints, poorer outcomes, higher staff sickness and attrition rates. Reducing staffing to save money is blinkered leadership, and every money-saving decision needs to be considered from a perspective that considers the impact on the quality of care and treatment.

---

59 NIHR (2019) *Having more registered nurses on general wards is linked to lower mortality* [online]. Available at: https://evidence.nihr.ac.uk/alert/having-more-registered-nurses-on-general-wards-is-linked-to-lower-mortality/ (accessed August 2023).

NHS England has an Impact Framework intended for use by NHS Trusts, but which could well be adapted for other providers.[60] The underpinning principles can be applied regardless of the decision-making process used. These principles are:

1. Be clear about what you are trying to achieve and understand what changes.

2. There is no one absolute measure of value – focus on creating a good-enough account of value at a point in time.

3. Judgements of value can and should be made by those involved in the work, not just third-party 'objective' evaluators.

4. Involve stakeholders in defining and evaluating value at meaningful intervals.

5. Be honest about contribution and attribution.

6. Don't dismiss the elements of value which are harder to capture.

7. Keep it simple and transparent.

8. Focus on learning, not just accountability.

The Commission published a report, *Monitoring the Mental Health Act in 2021 to 2022*, which said that workforce issues and staff shortages meant that people were not getting the level or quality of care they had a right to expect, and the safety of patients and staff was being put at risk.[61] The report recognised that some providers were trying to mitigate staffing issues by ensuring a better skill mix of staff on duty and increasing in-house training requirements. Others were said to be seeking alternative solutions, such as employing ward managers and other professionals to substitute for nursing cover. The Commission took the view that this was having a detrimental effect on staff safety and wellbeing, with staff working under sustained pressure and having to take on responsibilities they may not have been qualified for.

---

60   www.england.nhs.uk/sustainableimprovement/impact-framework/ (accessed August 2023).

61   CQC (2022) *Monitoring the Mental Health Act in 2021 to 2022* [online]. Available at: www.cqc.org.uk/publications/monitoring-mental-health-act/2021-2022 (accessed August 2023).

Fit and proper staff

Care providers must only employ people who can provide care and treatment appropriate to their role. They must have strong recruitment procedures in place and carry out relevant checks such as on applicants' criminal records and work history.

Not only must providers employ sufficient suitably qualified and experienced staff; they must also make sure that they reduce the risk of anyone they employ presenting a risk to the people they are treating or caring for. That, of course, is not just their health and social care staff but also their estates staff, their security staff, their porters or laundry staff and any volunteers.

There are some fairly shocking statistics about assaults within the NHS. A joint report published in 2023 found that NHS Trusts recorded more than 35,000 cases of rape, sexual assault, harassment, stalking and abusive remarks between 2017 and 2022.[62] The data obtained during the investigations showed that patients are the main perpetrators of abuse in hospitals. Most incidents (58%) involved patients abusing staff, with patients abusing other patients the next most common type of incident (20%). And although more than 4,000 NHS staff were accused of rape, sexual assault, harassment, stalking, or abusive remarks towards other staff or patients in 2017-22, the investigation found that only 576 have faced disciplinary action. 4,000 may be a small percentage (0.33%) of the 1.2 million staff employed in NHS Trusts, but it is still far too high and may not be an entirely complete picture. It means that one member of staff in every three hundred has faced an accusation of sexual misconduct.

Recruitments checks aren't a complete solution. They only put barriers up for those where concerns have been raised previously. Often, inappropriate behaviours go unchallenged, and no action is taken by providers because of the lofty position of the perpetrator. In September 2021, two UK surgical trainees called for more recognition and awareness of sexual harassment, sexual assault, and rape in the surgical profession.[63] In response, some other female surgeons shared their own experiences and lent support to strengthen the trainees' voices. It resulted in an apology from the Royal College of Surgeons.

It's not an issue to ignore – although that often happens. Having a DBS check and pre-employment checks is critical, but it won't prevent those who have never faced censure from continuing their behaviours. Having a known

---

62   Psy.org (2023) *Investigation reveals "shocking" epidemic of sexual assault in the NHS* [online]. Available at: https://phys.org/news/2023-05-reveals-epidemic-sexual-assault-nhs.html (accessed August 2023).

63   Bagenal J & Baxter N (2022) Sexual misconduct in medicine must end. *The Lancet* **399** (10329). www.thelancet.com/journals/lancet/article/PIIS0140-6736(22)00316-6/fulltext Accessed 25.5.2023.

policy for responding when someone raises concerns is essential, but it isn't enough – it has to both be followed and be seen to have been followed. It's not just about staff 'banter' being misunderstood or overstated either. That is blaming the victim rather than the perpetrators and doesn't protect anyone except the person with poor behaviours.

In 2021, a former member of staff at a Northern Irish care home was jailed for twenty-four years for sexually assaulting elderly residents at work and a young family member at home.[64] Videos on his phone showed him sexually assaulting extremely vulnerable elderly residents in the care homes where he worked. He admitted six counts of sexual assault and three counts of sexual assault by penetration against elderly, female care home residents between June and October 2015.

Also in 2021, a paramedic who raped a patient in her own home and sexually assaulted another in the back of an ambulance was jailed for twenty-one years.[65] He was convicted of six sexual offences. At his trial, he was found guilty of the rape and sexual assault of two women, and two counts of sexual assault of a child under the age of thirteen, who was not a patient. Police believe his career choice was "influenced by the access to potentially vulnerable" people. Fortunately, in this case, the Ambulance Trust acted entirely appropriately and followed their own policy. They suspended him pending the full investigation, referred him to the police and subsequently dismissed him. Their action in this situation prevented more people being harmed. That is why it is important to have the correct recruitment processes (even if you think you know someone), to have a clear policy that is known to everyone and, perhaps most importantly, to have a culture where people feel safe raising concerns and questions about others, knowing that their concerns will be treated with respect and acted upon when necessary.

It is worth leaders and providers knowing that new legislation has been introduced to protect employees in the workplace. The Worker Protection (Amendment of Equality Act 2010) Bill received Royal Assent on 26 October 2023.[66] It places a proactive duty on employers to take all reasonable steps to prevent sexual harassment in the workplace. So how can providers prepare and adapt to ensure compliance with the new legislation?

Like most aspects of good governance and good leadership, it is about having the right culture in place and then the governance systems to demonstrate that the culture is not allowing unwanted harassment by

64 BBC (2021) *Man jailed for abusing girl and care home residents* [online]. Available at: www.bbc.co.uk/news/uk-northern-ireland-57771411 (accessed August 2023).

65 BBC (2021) *NHS East of England Ambulance Service paramedic jailed for sexual assault of patients* [online]. Available at: www.bbc.co.uk/news/uk-england-cambridgeshire-56039255 (accessed August 2023).

66 https://bills.parliament.uk/publications/49773/documents/2921 (accessed August 2023).

minimising the impact on employees. Mainly, it is about listening to staff and addressing inappropriate behaviour when it first becomes apparent. Danny might only be "having a laugh" or "teasing Fatima"; He might "mean no harm" by it, and everyone may know "it's just Danny". Fatima, however, probably does not want her bottom touched or discussion about her legs. She has a right to take the matter to tribunal and may get an uplift in any compensation awarded.

The provider must be able to show that they took all reasonable steps to prevent and address the unwanted and unprofessional behaviour. They need to:

- **Review policies.** Examine existing harassment, bullying, equal opportunity, and other relevant policies. Update them to include training on different harassment scenarios, including third-party harassment, and provide guidance on intervention and support for victims.

- **Establish reporting lines.** Providers need to ensure clear reporting mechanisms so that employees can report harassment confidently and safely, and preferably have a reporting process outside of their line management structure where there is direct access to HR expertise and support for the individual. For NHS Trusts, this will also be the Freedom to Speak Up Guardian, and providers will want to ensure that the guardian is accessible to staff, can intervene and ensure that senior staff are aware of the concerns, and can signpost the person raising concerns to the appropriate policies and support.

- **Identify risks.** Identify harassment risks based on specific roles and circumstances. Consider which roles interact with third parties, and in what environments, and think about how the risks can be heightened for those who work alone. Maybe ensure that when someone says they don't want to work with Danny that there is a discussion about why not. Listen to employees and ask for their input on potential control measures such as body cameras or CCTV. Have senior staff visit staff rooms and even changing rooms (when empty) to look at the posters or messages on display. Consider introducing discussions at one-to-one reviews, or holding focus groups for specific groups who are known to be at greater risk of receiving unwanted sexual advances.

- **Incident reporting.** Encourage formal reporting of harassment incidents so that if there is a pattern, it can be identified and acted upon. Ensure that there is feedback to the individual and wider feedback when action has been taken, so that staff know something will be done and they will not suffer detriment for raising concerns.

- **Staff surveys.** Ensure that harassment is included on staff surveys so that the extent of any problem can be seen – and also to allow anonymous reporting when people feel too unsafe to raise the matter formally.

Duty of candour

Providers must be open and transparent with people using services about their care and treatment. Should something go wrong, they must be honest and open about what has happened, provide support and apologise.

I need to start this section by saying that there are regulatory requirements about the duty of candour.[67] The Commission publishes comprehensive guidance for providers so they can be clear what the expectations are. All providers and all leaders need to demonstrate an understanding of the regulatory requirements and make sure their staff follow their organisational policy. It's not sufficient to simply mumble a grudging apology that talks of being sorry that people feel upset about their treatment or care. My husband does that and it infuriates me, making a relatively minor situation worse!

The importance of this Fundamental Standard can be best understood with a little reflective practice and thinking about how you might feel if offered a half-hearted apology without accepting any culpability – or, worse still, if you didn't receive an apology at all. I'm trying to remember my husband's last aberration. He runs every morning across the South Downs and has a collection of trainers in various states of wetness, grass-covering and worse. He tends to pile them up near the door when he arrives home. We end up with three or four pairs scattered across the rear hall tiles with bits of mud and grass all around them. I can generally live with that, but if we have people coming for supper, they might use the lavatory off the hall, particularly if we are lucky enough to be eating outside. The trainers and grass/mud droppings look a mess, so I ask him to move them. After several reminders and excuses about needing them the next morning, he throws them up the back stairs towards our bedroom.

A couple of hours later I go to change, in a bit of a rush, before people arrive. I forget about the trainers. That part of our house is old and quite dark. I step on the trainers, lose my balance, and stumble up a few stairs bruising my knee. I am not best pleased and make this known. If he had said he was sorry and should have put them away properly, and poured me a medicinal glass of wine, I might have moved on. Instead, he tells me I saw him throw them on the stairs after I'd been nagging and should have looked where I was going. He adds that I have two pairs of shoes lying on the bedroom floor. You can see this might not be the most effective way to resolve an issue.

Most people that complain about their care or treatment want honest answers and an apology. In serious cases, they want to stop others going

---

67   CQC (undated) *The duty of candour: guidance for providers* [online]. Available at: www.cqc. org.uk/sites/default/files/20210421%20The%20duty%20of%20candour%20-%20guidance%20 for%20providers.pdf (accessed August 2023).

through what they, or someone they love, have suffered. NHS Resolution provides a good, brief guide to handling complaints and concerns that would work well in all health and social care settings. I recommend that everyone reads it.[68] It is called 'saying sorry', and it recognises that apologising meaningfully when things go wrong is vital for everyone involved in an incident – including the patient, their family, carers, and the staff that care for them.

The CQC will prosecute for breaches of the statutory Duty of Candour, and that can be expensive. In 2020, the first prosecution of a hospital Trust for failing to be open and transparent with the bereaved family of a ninety-one-year-old woman resulted in a significant fine.[69] The patient died in hospital after suffering a perforated oesophagus during an endoscopy. The Commission took the NHS Trust to court under duty of candour regulations, accusing it of not being open with the patient's family about the death and not apologising in a timely way. The Trust admitted its failings and was fined £12,565. The patient's daughter eventually received a letter of apology, but she felt it lacked remorse. She said she still had many unanswered questions and found it "impossible to grieve."

It's hard losing someone we love, and even harder if we don't understand why they died and why mistakes occurred.

Display of ratings

The provider of your care must display their CQC rating in a place where users can see it. They must also include this information on their website and make our latest report on their service available to you.

This Fundamental Standard is intended to help people understand the quality of care provided, and to make choices about where they receive care. Most people in England will have driven past care homes, GP practices or hospitals with huge banners tied to the front of the building declaring they are 'Good' or 'Outstanding' – usually the higher the rating, the bigger the banner. In principle, it is a good idea to enable people to see what rating a service has, but in practice the latest rating may be quite old and not a reflection of the current quality of the service. For smaller services, where there is less data, it might be a snapshot of just one or two days and not truly reflective of the service overall. Smaller providers also tend to have far fewer records of evidence to supply, making the judgement more dependent on a site visit.

---

68 https://resolution.nhs.uk/wp-content/uploads/2017/07/NHS-Resolution-Saying-Sorry-Final.pdf Accessed 26.5.2023

69 Morris S (2020) *NHS trust fined for lack of candour in first prosecution of its kind* [online]. Available at: www.theguardian.com/society/2020/sep/23/nhs-trust-fined-lack-of-candour-first-prosecution-of-its-kind-plymouth (accessed August 2023).

That is changing, and in future inspections will take a far more risk-based approach. Ratings will be able to change more frequently to enable a more current reflection of the quality of the service or part of a service. It was previously the case that a whole core service had to be inspected before a rating could be changed, but the work of the maternity review team in 2023, as part of the post-Ockenden reviews of maternity safety, has seen a movement towards changing ratings for just the 'safe' and 'well-led' domains that are then aggregated anew with the ratings that were not reviewed. That might tip a previously 'Good'-rated service into the red, and this in turn might well impact on the individual hospital or Trust-wide rating.

The regulatory requirement is to display the current rating, and to leave up a banner displaying an out-of-date 'Good' rating when a service has been rerated as 'Requires Improvement' is unacceptable. The new approach will inevitably focus on the 'safe' domain, and breaches of regulations that map to this domain will limit overall ratings.

Part 3:
The Quality
Statements

Chapter 11: Learning culture

Quality Statement:

We have a proactive and positive culture of safety based on openness and honesty, in which concerns about safety are listened to, safety events are investigated and reported thoroughly, and lessons are learned to continually identify and embed good practices.

There are eight Quality Statements within the 'Safe' domain, and in this section of the book I will devote a chapter to each one. The first – around creating and sustaining a learning culture – is an area that many providers fall short on. They believe that they follow a process, but it is often a tokenistic gesture with minimal investigation and an unimaginative action plan that is buried in a file on a computer system somewhere. Inspection teams ask the provider's staff about incidents, and they cannot think of a single time when they have seen a change because of an incident being reported. When the inspectors look at the investigation record, they see only a few comments about human error, or an action that is so vague as to be useless.

Recent reports where there are 'Requires Improvement' or 'Inadequate' ratings for safety usually identify a failure to learn from incidents. Willows Care Home in Chester was inspected in January 2023, and rated as 'Requires Improvement'.[70] The report said:

"Systems to review accidents and incidents did not prevent the risk of harm. Records detailed the actions taken in response to specific events which occurred. However, there had been no recorded analysis for trends for a period of six months."

Similarly, Yew Tree Residential Care Home in Lincolnshire was inspected in October 2022 and rated 'Inadequate'.[71] The report said:

"People were at risk of harm as opportunities to learn from incidents and reduce future risk were missed. There was no evidence of learning from incidents. There had been no analysis or review of falls/incidents since May 2022. Accident analysis forms for June, July, August, and September 2022 were blank. Accident forms were missing, so we were unable to determine what incidents had occurred or what action had been taken to reduce the risk of reoccurrence."

---

70   CQC (2023) *Willows Care Home Inspection Report* [online]. Available at: https://api.cqc.org.uk/public/v1/reports/98a0be6f-f3d3-4848-ae8d-b25c9edd4a27?20230307130000 (accessed August 2023).

71   CQC (2023) *Yew Tree Residential Care Home Inspection Report* [online]. Available at: https://api.cqc.org.uk/public/v1/reports/329fa79b-ae4f-4e70-b85b-67e7679b32f7?20230504120000 (accessed August 2023).

Similar statements are seen in most reports where enforcement action is taken, regardless of the type of service.

There are several sections to this Quality Statement, and each bears proper consideration. To begin with, "a proactive and positive culture of safety based on openness and honesty" is a very hard thing to achieve. Often providers and leaders believe they have achieved it, but staff and people using the services think otherwise.

The Nuffield Trust produces a report on the safety culture in the NHS using their QualityWatch indicator, which uses data from the NHS staff survey.[72] The Trust says that "a good safety culture in healthcare is one that includes value and respect for diversity, strong leadership and teamwork, openness to learning, and staff who feel psychologically safe (an environment where each individual feels they will be treated fairly and compassionately if they speak up)." They talk about being accountable and responsible for being capable, conscientious and not engaging in unsafe behaviour. They also say that those staff should not be held accountable for system failures. They recognise that leaders should hear patients' and caregivers' concerns regarding defects which interfere with the delivery of safe care and promote improvements in safety.

The Nuffield Trust's data shows that, in 2021, only 57% of NHS staff felt that they had the equipment, supplies and materials to do their job. Less than 30% felt that there were enough staff to enable them to do their jobs properly. This was a decline of 11%, from 38% in 2020 to 27% in 2021. If providers do not ensure that there are adequate staff to do the work allocated to the service, then they are not supporting a safety culture. Even the most dedicated staff can only do so much.

An example – maternity care

The CCQ has recently been carrying out reviews of safety in maternity services across England, driven partly by the 2022 Ockenden Report into maternity care at Shrewsbury and Telford Hospital NHS Trust. The recommendations from that review included:

- Incident investigations must be meaningful for families and staff, and lessons must be learned and implemented in practice in a timely manner.
- Staff must be able to escalate concerns if necessary.
- All Trusts must maintain a clear escalation and mitigation policy where maternity staffing falls below the minimum staffing levels for all health professionals.
- Trust boards must have oversight of the quality and performance of their maternity services.
- Staff who work together must train together.

---

72 www.nuffieldtrust.org.uk/qualitywatch (accessed August 2023).

There were other recommendations, but it is clear from those above that at the time of the review, Shrewsbury and Telford NHS Trust did not have a culture of safety.

In addition to the Ockenden Report, the CQC published a survey of maternity services users in 2022 that showed a worsening of women's ability to get the help they felt they needed during pregnancy and childbirth.[73] The survey reported that the proportion of women and other pregnant people being given the help they needed when they contacted a midwifery team during antenatal care dropped from 74% in 2017 to 69% in 2022. Similarly, women were less likely to say they were 'always' able to get a member of staff to help them when they needed attention during labour and birth; 63% in 2022 compared with 65% in 2021 and 72% in 2019. That may not seem like a huge drop until you think about the numbers. A 9% drop since 2019 means over 62,521 live births and 2,500 stillbirths. An awful lot of women clearly felt that they or their babies were at risk during pregnancy and labour.

These two issues, along with the emerging concerns around East Kent Hospitals University NHS Foundation Trust (where closing the maternity unit was considered) led to a specialist team being set up to deliver reviews of safety and leadership in maternity services across the country.[74,75] The nationwide review was intended to show how services were delivering in the context of current challenges and what extra help they may need. The Commission wanted to give women and their families an up-to-date view of the quality of maternity care at their local hospitals, and to give hospitals an objective assessment of what they were doing well and where improvements were being made. The programme of inspections was also intended to help the understanding of what was working and to enable the dissemination of good practice.

I suspect, but cannot evidence, that most of the Trusts where there were maternity review inspections felt that they had a good safety culture, that they addressed staff concerns and that they planned resources to enable staff to deliver safe care. A good number of the reports from the maternity reviews are published and in the public domain. They do not show a widespread proactive safety culture, but they do show boards of Trusts and integrated care systems (ICS) who were surprised by the reports. That is possibly the most concerning aspect of all to emerge from the reviews; not that there was inadequate staffing in some units, not that there was insufficient and incomplete investigation and action to address incidents,

73 CQC (2023) *Maternity survey 2022* [online]. Available at: www.cqc.org.uk/publication/surveys/maternity-survey-2022 (accessed August 2023).

74 ITV News (2023) *Watchdog considered closing East Kent maternity unit at centre of baby deaths scandal* [online]. Available at: www.itv.com/news/meridian/2023-05-26/scandal-hit-maternity-units-rated-inadequate-by-health-watchdog (accessed August 2023).

75 CQC (2022) *Maternity inspection programme* [online]. Available at: www.cqc.org.uk/guidance-providers/news/maternity-inspection-programme (accessed August 2023).

and not that there were services were the units where staff did not feel listened to. Most concerning of all was that the leaders in these services were unaware of the issues that were found.

The James Paget University Hospitals NHS Foundation Trust in Great Yarmouth was rated as 'Requires Improvement' for safety and leadership of maternity services. The report on this service, published in May 2023, says:

"We were not assured that leaders always understood the challenges and issues within the service. Where there was evidence of understanding of the challenges facing the service, we did not see evidence that effective plans translated into tangible actions and improvements, particularly as some of the issues identified had existed for an extended period, and some had been identified at the previous inspection in 2018."

The report also says:

"Staff told us they understood the duty of candour. However, they were not always open and transparent, and did not always give women and families a full explanation if and when things went wrong. Managers told us there had only been one incident eligible for the duty of candour process in 2022. We saw evidence of a duty of candour discussion with a woman by telephone in August 2022… However, duty of candour should be applied when patient-safety incidents are classified as moderate or severe harm or death. We found between April and December 2022 there were twenty-three incidents reported as moderate in severity."

Clearly, there are still women who are left with uncertainties and half-truths. And while the unit might have changed significantly since I myself had my youngest child there over twenty years ago, I suspect there are still lovely midwives trying to support women and provide a positive experience of birthing. The failings in the safety culture are not down to individuals. Each staff member is accountable for their own practice and behaviours, for raising concerns where there are perceived risks, for building positive relationships and for owning their mistakes, but it is for the provider to ensure that they make this so easy that it almost happens by default.

A climate of confidence

Staff need to feel safe to raise concerns and be persuaded to do so knowing that their concerns will be respected and addressed, if necessary. They need to know that, if a mistake has been made, they can speak up immediately to try and prevent a serious incident, or quickly enough to minimise any harms. Where something has gone wrong and someone has suffered harm, they need to be confident that their leaders will be open with the person who has suffered harm (and their families) and involve them in any investigation. It's really not rocket science, although defensive providers and leaders do try to nuance responses to the letter of the law to reduce any risk of litigation. As an aside, apologies don't increase the risk of compensation claims; they tend to reduce them, and they are one part of an overall culture of being open to the idea that learning from mistakes can help to improve safety.[76]

The same basis of developing a learning culture applies whatever the type of service. Imagine a start-up domiciliary care agency with only three employees, plus the provider who is also the manager. One employee has a rota that requires her to drive to support Mrs Smith to get up and have some breakfast. Mrs Smith lives on Lyndhurst Avenue. Now imagine the care support worker is rushing as she has a child who is unwell, and she had to arrange emergency childcare. She glances at her list and mistakenly sees that she is down to help Mr Smith (who she has visited many times before, and who lives on Lynmouth Road). She goes to see Mr Smith, who is a bit surprised to see someone from the agency as his daughter was due to arrive any moment and no care visit was planned for the day.

The care worker looks at her list again and realises her error. She calls the manager in a panic. Poor Mrs Smith is still in bed and probably hungry. The manager says it's too late now to go to her, and instead to carry on with the other clients. Mrs Smith will have the community nurse going in shortly, and the manager can ring and say Mrs Smith was uncooperative and refused to be helped. The manager also shouts at the care worker for being stupid and says she will lose an hour's pay as she didn't make the visit. The worker uses the team WhatsApp to tell the other carers, as she is so upset.

Based on these events, are the other care staff likely to say if they make a mistake? Will the manager's response reduce the risk of a similar mistake occurring in the future? If the community nurse goes in and find Mrs Smith on the floor, cold, and clearly having passed away some hours previously, what will she most likely do? Does anyone benefit from not owning mistakes and not responding appropriately? If you were Mrs Smith's son, would you forgive a member of staff arriving an hour late more readily than a lie about a visit being refused that left your mother dead?

Evidence to support the Quality Statement

So, how can you evidence this Quality Statement to demonstrate that you are meeting the required standards?

Inspections of services using the single assessment framework are based on evidence from three different source types. Providing information against each type is likely to demonstrate more readily that you have considered and met the requirements for a 'Good' rating, at least. If you have all the

---

76 https://www.med.stanford.edu/news/all-news/2017/10/in-patient-injury-cases-offering-apology-does-not-lead-to-lawsuit-increase.html (accessed August 2023).

evidence and give it to the inspection team, then it is easier for them to see what you have achieved. Ideally, you will be able to provide 1) evidence from people using the service, 2) evidence from staff and 3) data and records-based evidence.

The third area – data, records and paperwork – is the easiest to provide evidence for and should be your most reliable source over time. Staff and service users are human beings, and any given individual may not have a full picture of a situation.

Evidence from data and records

Provider or unit records are an important way of demonstrating that concerns are genuinely listened to and acted upon in practice. How that is done is provider-dependent, and the Commission cannot tell services how they must record and investigate concerns. Nor can they 'mark them down' if those records are not kept and presented in a format that a particular inspector prefers. If that were to happen, it would be worthy of a challenge at the factual accuracy stage.

Of course, services that provide care and treatment under NHS contracts are required to use the NHS Patient Safety Incident Response Framework (PSIRF).[77] NHS England have allowed a twelve-month period for organisations to prepare for the transition to PSIRF, with an expected timescale for completion by autumn 2023. During this preparation phase, organisations must continue using the current Serious Incident Framework.[78] During any inspection involving the 'well-led' key question, or a 'well-led' inspection of a Trust, providers offering NHS services (not just NHS Trusts, but also independent providers contracting with the NHS) are likely to be asked about their preparations, their rollout plans and any mitigation of risk when moving from one framework to another. Those plans need to be operational rather than strategic. They must be visible, and they must demonstrate forward movement.

An electronic action plan with all actions flagging green would be a good way to evidence that the changes were being delivered in a planned, progressive manner. Maybe this could be shared regularly with the Commission via the portal or during engagement meetings. I think it's probably important to realise that the provider-based senior staff are likely to be more knowledgeable about the transition to the new framework than many of the CQC staff, as while inspectors will retain their sector-specific role, operations managers and leaders will not and may have a background

---

77 www.england.nhs.uk/wp-content/uploads/2020/08/200312_Introductory_version_of_Patient_Safety_Incident_Response_Framework_FINAL.pdf (accessed August 2023).

78 www.england.nhs.uk/wp-content/uploads/2020/08/serious-incidnt-framwrk.pdf (accessed August 2023).

in adult social care, primary medical services or delivery and performance. Sharing in a way that allows the Commission staff to understand what you are doing has to be a good thing for both parties, and it may fall to providers to take the initiative.

Incident reporting and investigation

All services need an incident reporting and investigation policy – no matter how small the service, or how well a tiny team is perceived to communicate. Hopefully it won't happen, but if you were taken to court or a coroner's hearing, could you demonstrate that you had followed your policy? There is a well-worn adage in the CQC that if it isn't recorded, then it didn't happen. You can tell an inspection team (or a court) until you are blue in the face that everyone knew what was expected and that staff knew how to raise concerns, but without a current policy nobody is going to accept that. A policy is the starting point of good incident management. It may well be bureaucratic nonsense and something you haven't got time for, but when something goes wrong it becomes vitally important. Probably best to err on the side of caution and have a policy in place before things go wrong as – not least because, correctly applied, a good reporting and investigation policy can actually stop things from going wrong.

The policy must be current. I recall a hospice that moved from premises that were no longer fit for purpose to a beautiful new building. Six months later, they still hadn't updated many of their policies. Few incidents were being formally recorded, and there were several complaints about a lack of privacy as the footpath from the car park to the main reception was immediately alongside the bedrooms. Staff knew about this before complaints started appearing, but they were unsure of how to raise it as the staffing structure, the reporting systems and the escalation routes had all changed. Nobody thought to tell the staff how to actually bring about change in their new world.

This hospice provider is a very good provider, and the staff pride themselves on giving high-quality, proactive, personalised care. They responded to the complaints swiftly, moved the path and added private terraces and garden areas to the bedrooms, allowing patients and their families time together in a lovely outdoor setting. The gardening volunteers made sure that each garden was well-maintained and offered year-round interest, with bird song and the scent of roses or a bright display of newly emerged snowdrops. Unfortunately for the three families who complained, they felt their loved one died without privacy and that they had had to endure people staring in at them in their final days. That can't be undone.

Apologies help, and explanations of improvements made also help, but had the provider made sure that the staff knew how to raise concerns easily, they might have made the changes before anyone suffered the indignity of dying in view of others.

There are policies available to purchase. Sometimes, staff bring a copy of their previous employer's policy with them, or there is a corporate policy. There is nothing wrong with any of those options if the staff and leadership team have worked through the policy and made sure it is both workable and applicable to their settings. It is no use plagiarising a policy from GP practice where your registered manager used to work if it talks about electronic reporting and speaking to a partner, and the current service has no electronic system and no partners. By all means take a draft policy, even the NHS England one, but make it provider- and service-specific.

Make sure that the policy makes clear to staff what needs reporting, along with how and when. A concern about a trip hazard in a care home reported three weeks later when the registered manager remembers to update the incident book may result in a serious injury to a resident. Also make sure that any mention of safeguarding referrals (which there should be) refer to the correct local authority. And ensure that the policy links to other relevant policies including the safeguarding policy, the Medicines Management Policy, the Response to Allegations of Inappropriate Behaviour policy, the Equality and Diversity policy and any others that are relevant to the setting and type of services being delivered.

The policy needs to be updated at regular intervals – even if there are no changes, it needs to be checked, and that check must be recorded and a new review date set. This is particularly so if the policy links closely to another provider's policy, as that other provider's policy may well have changed in the interim.

On the subject of policies linking to umbrella policies, it is important to remember that the regulations apply to each provider. Therefore, each provider needs its own policy. An independent emergency ambulance provider that contracts exclusively with an NHS Ambulance Trust cannot simply say, "We use the Ambulance Trust policy." They may well feed into the Ambulance Trust governance systems, but they also need to have their own systems and that starts with a policy. That policy might say that the independent ambulance provider crews are to report patient-related incidents to the Hospital Ambulance Liaison Officer (HALO) at the hospital where they have taken the patient, and that they need the Datix number for the incident so the provider can follow up with the NHS Ambulance Trust to ensure that appropriate action was taken, and the incident can be closed. However, the independent ambulance provider will still need their own reporting system, because not all incidents are patient related. A crash into a car park bollard is nothing to do with an NHS Ambulance Trust, is it?

A policy is no use if it is printed out, covered in coffee cup rings, and stuck in a drawer when someone decided to tidy the office. So, what should you do with it?

Villages and volunteers – a personal story

My husband and I met after our A-levels, when we spent a summer (and many more afterwards) taking disadvantaged children from more challenged areas of London on holidays to villages in the countryside or by the seaside. We started as enthusiastic and naïve teenagers, but were always kind, and we knew how to have fun and how to allow children to have fun, with a nod to safety. As we developed professional understanding, we realised that the charity needed to modernise, and that some sort of governance was required to ensure that the thousands of children sent on holiday each year were offered safe care. There were some fairly high-risk practices that, within a year or two of starting professional training, my then-boyfriend, now husband, and I realised had to change if we were to remain working with the charity.

At a meeting with the General Secretary to discuss this, we asked whether there were any childcare policies, any guidance for host families (yes, children were sent to private homes for two weeks with minimal checks) or volunteers on the camps. She coughed loudly, stubbed out her cigarette and started rummaging in her desk. Then she opened the office door and bellowed at the administrator. Bellowing was her default setting; she was very loud, although she wasn't unkind. The administrator arrived with a couple of sheets of paper stuck together with a slice of pepperoni pizza. Reading what wasn't obliterated with grease, we determined that it focused on how host families could arrange for children to be moved if they were unsuitable in some way. This was the sum total of their policies and governance. We continued to work with the charity for a decade, but during that time I was commissioned to write a schedule of policies and operating protocols. Times had moved on, and the charity needed to modernise and show it met current acceptable standards.

I include this story as, having written the polices and agreed them with the Trustees, they could easily have been put back under the pizza and not seen the light of day until something bad happened. Instead, we worked with the charity to introduce training based on the policies and protocols for cap volunteers, to ensure that copies of the volunteer handbook (based on the policies) were posted to all London and country-based volunteers, and to set up a governance programme that involved benchmarking visits to all the summer camps and a feedback questionnaire for volunteers and for families who had sent children to camp. It wasn't perfect, and some troubling incidents could still slip through, but it was a big step towards the charity accepting accountability for what was happening to the children they sent on holiday.

The introduction of standard policies, recruitment practices and training was not universally popular. Some very established camp leaders said it was trying to make a voluntary role professional, and some groups who hosted summer camps didn't want to be told what to do since they had fundraised and staffed the camps themselves. We stuck firm, and a newly appointed CEO supported us. And, on the whole, the volunteer supervisors loved the training weekends and said they felt much more confident managing behaviours and the needs of individual children afterwards.

The visits found some really lovely holidays taking place, but also picked up a variety of concerns. One group took a coach load of seven to twelve-year-old children to camp in their rural village. They had a great programme of activities and outings, and the food provided by the local WI was amazing, but they hadn't got particularly good shower facilities (in fact, only one staff shower), so they farmed the children out for a couple of 'pamper evenings' in the homes of local people. Those evenings involved a nice meal, warm fluffy towels and their kindly hosts bathing the children. The group said the vicar knew all the hosts personally, so they knew the children would be treated well. I'm sure most of the hosts were lovely, but the risk was too high for the children. Having a current agreed policy meant that the CEO could simply say to the volunteers that this was against charity policy and that it had to stop, or no children would be sent to the village in future years. Having a ratified policy means that staff and others can be held to account and required to conform to expected standards.

Storage and retrieval of policies

At this point, it might be worth thinking about how you store and, more importantly, view or retrieve policies for the service. Policies need to be visible and known to be used. Providers and managers need to ensure that they can demonstrate that staff have read and understood the policy in order to hold them to account, if necessary. If the organisational policy is that staff must check water temperatures before using a hoist to lower residents into baths, but someone ends up badly scalded because a staff member didn't check the temperature, who is at fault here? It might seem that any sensible person puts their hand in and feels the bath temperature before lowering somebody into the water. However, that is not how culpability and responsibility work.

If the provider had ensured that, as part of induction, the staff member was required to sign to say they had read and understood the policy, and they still lowered somebody into scalding water, then they would have to accept a degree of responsibility; if they are professionally registered, they might face censure from their professional body or even a court. If the provider can demonstrate that all staff must read the policy and sign to say they understand it, that there are water thermometers in each bathroom and that they keep records of bath temperature checks, then the individual staff member is going to find it hard to argue that they thought all water was thermostatically controlled. Ideally, of course, water to baths and showers would be thermostatically controlled, but that is a separate issue.

The importance of trends

So, the documentary and written evidence required for the 'learning culture' Quality Statement to receive a tick on inspection day is:

- A current, ratified written policy relating to incident reporting, investigation, and mitigation of future risk.
- A record that staff have read and understood the policy. That means all staff.
- Some evidence that staff are trained and reminded to follow the policy.
- A recording system appropriate to the type of service and nature of care and treatment being provided.
- A record of the investigations and action taken to prevent recurrence. If you can demonstrate the ongoing effectiveness of that action, so much the better.
- A record of how feedback was given to the person reporting the incident.
- Details of how the learning was shared across the team or wider organisation, if necessary. Some incidents don't necessarily have much learning (a flat tyre, for example), but most do.
- Evidence (probably in the recording and investigation record) that links to other policies, such as safeguarding, have been considered for each incident.
- Evidence that the Duty of Candour has been considered and applied, when necessary.

As can be seen from several of the items on this list, a key aspect of meeting this Quality Statement is providing evidence that the service identifies trends or themes and acts on them. In order for that to happen, there needs to be a culture where incidents and near misses are recorded. You cannot, after all, audit or review an incident that has not been entered on the system you use. In small services, that review might simply be working through the incident log (paper or electronic) and coding them (just a word – maybe Medicines – or different coloured highlighters with a key to the colours on the side), to highlight anything that looks like a pattern. If a basic pattern is identified, then more digging may be needed to understand what is going on – not an onerous task for smaller organisations, and if an Excel-based system is used in slightly larger organisations, then it can be filtered very easily.

In May 1991 Beverly Allitt, an enrolled paediatric nurse, was arrested for the murders of four children and the attempted murders of nine others who were being cared for on a children's ward. She was found guilty and moved to Rampton Secure Hospital, where she remains. The Independent Inquiry acknowledged that it was sometimes very difficult to stop someone set on grievous acts, but also made recommendations to try to mitigate future risks to young patients.[79] A key consideration was whether swifter action and a review of the unexpected child injuries and deaths had any commonality, any pattern. Allitt was eventually caught when police looked in detail at which staff were on duty when the deaths occurred. There was a pattern, but it wasn't seen in time to prevent the murder and attempted murder of thirteen children.

Much more recently, in August 2023, Lucy Letby, a neonatal nurse, was prosecuted for the murder of seven babies and the attempted murder of six other infants. Letby is only the third woman alive to be given a whole life sentence; she will never leave prison and will serve her time in one of three restrictive custody centres. It is very difficult to pre-judge the learning before publication of the report from the statutory public inquiry, which is being led by Lady Justice Thirwall – one of the most senior Court of Appeal judges. There is also still a possibility of a retrial for the attempted murder of six babies where the jury could not reach a verdict. It would be wrong to linger on the possible outcomes of either a retrial or the public inquiry. That said, we know that that police are reviewing the care and treatment of a further four thousand babies admitted to the neonatal units where Letby worked, and that the Parliamentary and Health Service Ombudsman has called for the public inquiry remit to be widened to consider whether there is a wider NHS culture of covering up patient safety and care failings.

I imagine most leaders, managers and healthcare professionals have been both saddened and horrified by the case. That a neonatal nurse would harm the infants in her care is almost beyond belief, and yet the evidence was compelling enough that she was given a whole life term. Hopefully, even before publication of the report every hospital leader, every nurse, every doctor, every person caring for the vulnerable will be asking whether it could happen in their workplace. I imagine the initial reaction will be "No, definitely not". I would also hope that a deeper consideration would look at not whether but how it could – and more importantly how the service can protect those it looks after. Of course, working for the regulator I have wondered whether we could have been more proactive in monitoring neonatal outcomes, whether we should have spotted the trend. My conclusion is that I do not know enough about the data we held and the monitoring of the specific providers to make a fair judgement about that.

I would hope that, moving forward, staff are being listened to and that their concerns and questions are not dismissed as too unlikely to be taken seriously. We need to remind ourselves that Lucy, the nurse (rather than Letby, the serial killer) was perceived as lovely, gentle and smiley. Ian

79 Clothier C (1994) *The Allitt inquiry: independent inquiry relating to deaths and injuries on the children's ward at Grantham and Kesteven General Hospital during the period February to April 1991.* London: HMSO, 1994.

Paterson the rogue breast surgeon was similarly said to be charismatic and charming. The other key lesson that must come from this tragedy is understanding trends and themes that the data is showing us, and looking for the possibility of correlation between and causes of coincidences.

Of course, the likelihood of finding a killer on your wards or in your service is very low. What is more likely is that the incidents show that perhaps one nurse makes more medicines errors than anyone else and might need support to become more competent, or that the times of the drugs rounds are when several staff have breaks and so the nurse is torn between answering bells and handing out medicines. It might be that an ambulance is sometimes left unstocked or dirty after one particular paramedic has been driving, or it might be that several staff voice concerns about the behaviour of a particular GP who never uses chaperones. A good provider will review their data (incident records) to see if there are patterns. The larger providers will want, I hope, to be reviewing their incident data for wider patterns and for benchmarking – one care home reporting far more pressure damage or falls than others in the group, perhaps, or a maternity unit where the time taken to answer triage calls has increased over time and where women are hanging up more frequently.

Action planning

Action plans can be a useful way of providing evidence of action when incidents are reported. I say 'can', because they often offer evidence of a lack of learning and support the idea that nothing has changed. There are providers where the same incidents are reported over and over again, and the action plans are a literal 'cut and paste' of previous, very similar incidents with minimal thought and minimal evidence of effective action or organisational learning. Let's consider a hypothetical example:

A grade-three pressure wound in a care home is reported as an incident. It is the third such wound that the home has reported, and a safeguarding referral should also have been made but wasn't. The care home clinical lead carries out the investigation and creates an action plan that is the same for each of the incidents reported. All report that the wounds were attributable to the people being incontinent and having reduced mobility. The action plan says simply 'staff to check that care plans are followed'. That won't prevent further pressure damage incidents, will it?

Action plans need to be sufficient to reduce the risk of recurrence. It is good practice to ensure that they are suitable for organisational learning, and also good to practice them in case you are asked to submit an action plan after an inspection. The CQC staff monitoring the response should be checking whether the action plan submitted by providers is sufficient to address the shortfalls.

The Parliamentary and Health Service Ombudsman has produced guidance on action planning, which is very useable in all settings.[80] It is very simple and offers templates and a checklist. Action planning isn't complicated; we all do it consciously and subconsciously in many aspects of our life. Planning a wedding is action planning by another name, as is arranging a camping trip in France or moving house. We don't always write it down in action-plan format, but the thought process is very similar. Action planning obviously comes after identifying root causes. It then needs clarity about who will do what, when and how, with detail about resources, timescales, measures of success and who is responsible for what bits. There also needs to be a monitoring process included as part of the plan, so that it can be reviewed and amended if it isn't bringing about the desired changes.

An action plan should be a live tool, not something left unseen and unchanged. It needs to have someone who is responsible for implementation and monitoring. If you were planning a summer fete, you wouldn't just expect everyone to turn up and do their bit, would you? You'd have someone in charge, or a committee overseeing the arrangements. If that committee saw that the weather forecast had changed, and torrential rain and thunderstorms were expected, they might want to revisit the plans for afternoon tea in the garden and the Morris dancing display. Similarly, the third incident of a grade-three pressure wound should make the registered manager or leader of a service question whether the action plan was effective and consider what else might be needed and whether the monitoring arrangements were adequate.

Evidence from staff and service users

Evidence from staff

So, if a provider has good data and records, what further evidence might come from staff to reinforce the impression that this is a high-quality service? The documentary requirements and proper use of incident reports go a long way to ensuring that staff provide useful evidence that supports a view that a service is compliant.

You cannot tell staff what to say, but you can support them to feel confident when an inspection team appears – a 'rabbit in the headlights' look suggests a lack of knowledge or confidence, even if that isn't the case and the staff member simply feels a huge personal responsibility for the outcome of the inspection. Even seemingly strong and confident senior leaders can get flustered. Having built a strong safety culture (or at least being on the road towards that point) means that staff can answer questions and provide examples when asked. If you coach them well, they can offer up their own

---

80 www.ombudsman.org.uk/organisations-we-investigate/putting-things-right/writing-action-plans (accessed August 2023).

relevant examples rather than waiting to be asked. Just don't have everyone give exactly the same, identically worded example (unless this was about something discussed in a very recent team meeting).

Don't fudge or apply pressure to 'say the right thing'. Most inspectors can see through half-truths and learned words. If providers and leaders have the right attitudes and have built a good culture, the staff will say this. That is what you're aiming for.

Evidence from people for this Quality Statement is likely to be around staff being asked about learning from incidents and changes made in response to any risks identified. They will be asked whether they feel happy raising concerns and, if they simply say "Yes", they may be asked to give examples. Sometimes, it can seem like pulling teeth, trying to get staff to talk to the inspection team about examples where they've raised concerns and what has been done about it. But in many cases, this is simply because the language they and the inspection team use isn't always aligned.

For example, telling a fleet manager that a warning light has come on in Ambulance 3 may just feel to the member of staff as if they are telling the boss the vehicle needs looking at. They may not think of it as 'raising a concern', but it is. And if the fleet manager comes back to the driver and says he's taken it off the road to be looked at, and to use Ambulance 2 instead, then that is action and feedback. Yet because the staff member doesn't see it like that, they may give the all-too-frequent blank look when the inspector asks about any feedback from raising concerns.

Staff need to understand that informing relevant people about issues is 'raising concerns' and being told what is happening is 'feedback'. Managers and leaders can support this by using appropriate language. In our scenario, maybe the fleet manager could say "Thanks, Shara, please can you write it as a concern in the incident log before we all forget?" Then instead of simply saying, "Use Ambulance 2, for now", he might say "Use Ambulance 2 for now, and once I've spoken with the garage, I'll send you a feedback email to let you know what the problem was". This way, the language of inspection is learned without staff even thinking about it. And, when an inspector subsequently asks whether they've ever reported a concern and if so whether they had feedback, it will be much easier for the staff member to recall the warning light.

A really well-versed leader (not only the registered manager or an executive, but maybe a departmental head or member of a triumvirate), would be able to talk about how their service supports staff to report incidents via whatever method is in place. In NHS services the staff will use Datix, the electronic reporting and management system – but it doesn't matter what the system is, as long as there is one.

How do you turn everyday occurrences into 'evidence'? The key lies in helping staff understand that this is what it is. For a large provider, it might be that this is done at local unit level, in team meetings. A ward manager might run through the log of concerns raised and what has been done about them at a team meeting. Some places have a 'you said, we did' noticeboard for staff. While in isolation these things may not be sufficient, they are part of embedding the language and process of 'concerns' and 'feedback' in the minds of staff. Make sure it is both current and talked about. Certainly, all serious incidents should be shared widely, along with any details of immediate actions or changes and any longer-term mitigations.

Some larger providers do glossy newsletters around incidents and actions. This helps staff understand what learning there is, and to see that reporting concerns means that things get done. Small providers may not have the funds for this, but a regular email update or a box on the governance team's newsletter can be a useful way of sharing learning from incidents and building a safety culture.

So, what do staff say the reasons for not reporting incidents are? Why are some incidents not investigated? varies enormously. If I had to list them, I might say:

- **Challenges in reporting incidents.** Making reporting easy makes it more likely. Access to the reporting system during work hours is often a stumbling block – staff may have to get someone to unlock an office where an incident book is kept or go to another part of the premises to write in a book or fill in a spreadsheet.

- **Not believing it makes a difference.** Low staffing is often an issue here. Then, when an inspection team arrives, they hear that the service is understaffed, that leaders have been informed and nothing has been done. This is where feedback is always a winner – not only do staff know they can influence how the service is delivered and that risks are considered, but they also know they are listened to. Feedback may not mean three more nurses on every shift, but it might be a sharing of how dependency and staffing are reviewed, and any risks addressed.

- **A feeling that they will be criticised for reporting incidents.** A culture of toxic positivity where leaders only want to hear good-news stories, and where problems are dismissed and hidden from senior leaders for fear of criticism and damage to the organisation's reputation. Raising concerns can be prejudicial to people's careers and people voicing concerns (particularly about the behaviours of peers or leaders), can be seen as troublemaking.

- **A lack of recording.** An absence of records of how incidents are investigated and learned from usually occurs because investigations aren't done at all or aren't done well. This can be a costly mistake. It doesn't enhance reputations if it is reported on, and it can be costly if a pattern was there to be seen but not looked for.

Providers who make it easy for staff to report incidents, and who ensure that staff understand the importance of doing so, are likely to have staff who tell inspection teams about the incident process. Even better if the provider is very clear about any leadership, system or resource shortfalls, and makes sure that the investigation doesn't just put mistakes down to human failings or, worse, blame and censure staff. Of course, if a member of staff consciously provides poor care, is unkind, fails to follow policy repeatedly or acts outside their level of competence, then addressing that is important. What you shouldn't do is say that is the entire problem.

Imagine that you are the manager of the operating theatre in a private hospital; four theatres each running a different theatre list, two with orthopaedic lists every day except Sunday. Usually, you only run two morning lists and two afternoon lists, but the provider has taken on a large new NHS contract to help the local system manage their waiting list backlog. You had mentioned that this was asking a lot of staff to the hospital director, and pointed out that there were already a few operating department practitioner (ODP) vacancies and recovery nurse vacancies, plus there were no trained children's nurses and the hospital director was offering some ear, nose and throat surgery to children over five years of age. Your role is currently a secondment, and you want a permanent role at the same level, and you don't want to jeopardise your career, so when you are told that you need to make it work, you say you will.

You use an agency nurse in recovery who used to work on the ward, so knows the hospital and the policies. She offers to work long days (7am– 7pm) on her days off from her care home job each week, to help with the rising cost of living. She has two children of her own, so she understands children – although she is a bit nervous about children in recovery. You tell her it's only ENT surgery and is part of the role – if she can't do it then another agency nurse will. A four-year-old child becomes very unwell following a tonsillectomy. They deteriorate quickly and the agency nurse doesn't spot it as there is no paediatric early warning tool in use. The child had probably started off swallowing copious amounts of blood. She calls for help and an ODP tells her the anaesthetist has already left as the last patient was out of theatre. The ODP bleeps the resident medical officer and the senior nurse on duty. They manage to stabilise the child sufficiently to transfer them to a local NHS hospital and then onwards to a children's hospital with a critical care unit.

How many lessons are there and for whom? Where does culpability sit? What are the root causes? What might an action plan look like? How does that agency nurse feel, do you think? What would the feedback to her be? What about the child's parents? What are they told and what support should they receive? This may seem a bit of an extreme example, but it is based quite closely on a real situation.[81] It might be a useful exercise to imagine this in your service, and to think whether your incident processes would support learning from a similar incident. What do you do when staff raise a concern or share a mistake? How do leaders behave, and how are staff encouraged to share that mistake to reduce the risk of others doing something similar?

Evidence from service users

The next thing to consider is how you might provide evidence about raising concerns from people using services. How easy that is will vary depending on the service type and how many people are using the service at the time of any inspection. Sometimes there are barely any service users for inspection teams to speak to, and sometimes the team can speak to lots of people. Often the conversations are a bit limited and revolve around whether people say they would be happy to voice concerns or raise a complaint. This is a bit colourless. Providers and leaders can make it easier for the inspection team to gather evidence from people using services about incidents and raising concerns, although it crosses over into the documents/records section, perhaps.

Just as any inspection team should stop at the end of an inspection and ask whether the provider or local leaders are happy with the way an inspection has been conducted, so too providers or leaders might want to add a step at the end of an incident investigation record that asks the people involved whether they are happy with the way the incident has been handled and their involvement. That might be the member of staff reporting the incident, people using services or their families. The ways in which a registered manager, a provider or a local leader can seek feedback from service users are too numerous to list in full here, but might include:

- **A verbal question.** Often matrons in private hospitals walk around each day and ask each patient if they are happy with their care and the service they have received. When inspectors ask about raising concerns, many will say that matron comes around every day. In an NHS hospital, the Chief Nurse obviously cannot visit every patient every day, but they can ask the unit matrons, the ward sisters or department leaders to speak to each person using their part of a service.

- **Personal visits.** As part of incident-reporting governance, representatives of the board and provider can visit various parts of an organisation and ask if staff and people using the service feel able to voice concerns and are encouraged to report incidents. Staff should be asked whether they have done so and, if they have, whether they received feedback. These 'walk-around visits' are quite informal,

---

81 BBC News (2013) *Child surgery stopped over 'life-threatening' failings at Mount Alvernia Hospital* [online]. Available at: www.bbc.com/news/uk-england-surrey-22379133 (accessed August 2023).

usually, but should be recorded – date, time, name of person visiting, number of staff and service users spoken to, the number who were specifically asked about raising concerns and reporting incidents, and their responses.

- **Audits and reviews** of incident reporting and investigations should consider whether the process had involved the people affected, whether the duty of candour has been met and whether there has been any feedback to the person raising concerns. Gaps in any of these considerations should be addressed.

- **Local surveys.** I would want to know what service users, their families and my staff felt about a service I ran. Part of that would be offering a chance to provide feedback, and asking about their confidence to voice concerns or mention risks.

- **Healthwatch.** A positive, proactive relationship with your local Healthwatch can be invaluable. Inviting them in for a voluntary 'enter and view' visit will give lots of independent insight and fresh eyes. They might get feedback from people who have questions or concerns and don't feel able to raise them with the provider. I would want to know if someone I was providing care or treatment to didn't think they could talk to me or someone from my service if things went wrong.

- **Service user or relatives' meetings** don't happen often in the NHS anymore. As a staff nurse in charge at a weekend, I used to make a huge pot of tea, put out some biscuits and have all the parents who wanted to talk sit around a table in the biggest bay on the ward. Sometimes we discussed the weather, but now and then an individual would be emboldened enough by the informality and the presence of others to say they were worried about something or had noticed a problem. Once it was that the wire mesh on the balcony, where little children often played and waved to people, had a hole in it and they were worried a child might be able to get through. A quick glance showed that the parent was right – a hole had appeared and the gap between the railings was just large enough for a four-year-old to squeeze through. They might not have mentioned it without our Sunday meetings, which put parents and staff on a more equal footing.

Freedom to Speak Up Guardians support workers to speak up when they feel that they are unable to in other ways.[82] This is a statutory requirement in the NHS, and there are over 900 Freedom to Speak Up Guardians in the NHS and among independent sector organisations, national bodies and elsewhere. The National Guardian's Office leads the national network of Freedom to Speak Up Guardians in England and provides support and challenge to the healthcare system on speaking up. Integrated care boards

---

82 https://nationalguardian.org.uk/ (accessed August 2023).

should have oversight of the Freedom to Speak Up Guardians in all the NHS services in their area. It is recommended that each Integrated Care System appoints an executive and non-executive lead for Freedom to Speak Up to provide leadership for this.

Some large adult social care providers have begun to introduce Freedom to Speak Up Guardians, as have some private healthcare providers (particularly those with NHS contracts). The National Guardians Office provides training resources and case studies to support the growth of the Freedom to Speak Up movement. And Freedom to Speak Up Guardians don't have to be limited to NHS organisations or private healthcare providers who contract with NHS services. There is nothing to stop care home providers or domiciliary care providers offering a similar service. If the Guardian sits outside the line-management structure, or is fully independent but with access to senior staff and board members, then so much the better.

Chapter 12: Safe systems, pathways and transitions

Quality Statement:

We work with people and our partners to establish and maintain safe systems of care, in which safety is managed, monitored, and assured. We ensure continuity of care, including when people move between different services.

This Quality Statement is about governance, and it includes the responsibilities of the duty of candour and acting on complaints. It is also about safe care and treatment, as all the Quality Statements are, and how providers work together to ensure that there is continuity of care when moving between services.

In terms of regulatory processes, looking at transitions can present challenges around determining where the responsibility sits for any care shortfalls or increased risk. Care and treatment delivery is often shared across providers and can have the involvement of many health and social care services, which means there must be greater consideration of the pathway and how the moves between different parts of it can be made seamless. There are some excellent examples of this working when the commitment is there, and it is often when the need is most pressing that providers and staff find ways to come together to provide exceptional care in difficult circumstances.

There are plenty of good examples of planning and commissioning of services to provide easier transitions. Sussex Community NHS Foundation Trust provides the 'ECHO' service that improves the coordination and delivery of end-of-life care across the coastal areas of West Sussex by linking key services via a 24/7 telephone hub staffed by trained nurses. The service sees a number of providers working closely together for the benefit of the patients and their families, including Sussex Community NHS Foundation Trust, Western Sussex Hospitals NHS Foundation Trust, Macmillan Cancer Support, St Barnabas House, and St Wilfrid's Hospice, Chichester. That means they have shared working with the acute hospitals, the two adult hospices in the area (who also offer hospice at home, day hospice and Community Palliative Care Teams), the community nursing service, and support services from a voluntary organisation. People who are approaching the end of their life and their families just have to call one number to access all the support they need.

There are also lots of concerns raised about the way patients are discharged from hospital without the necessary support being arranged, or about those who fall through gaps between services. Hospitals are under huge pressure to clear backlogs, and to move those people who are medically fit for discharge from hospital to free up beds for admissions. Doing that safely requires planning and monitoring to ensure that the plans are activated, and that the carers that have been arranged do actually turn up to provide the support that people need. A delayed transfer of care occurs when a patient is medically fit for discharge but must stay in hospital for non-medical reasons. Common issues which cause delays include a lack of suitable equipment at home, unavailability of community care packages, and waiting for a bed in a residential or nursing home to become available.

Not planning for discharge is expensive. A recent systematic review reported that delayed discharges cost between £200 and £565 per patient, per day.[83] Analysis by Age UK in 2019 estimated that delayed discharge due to unavailability of social care support cost the country £640,000 per day.[84] Hospitals now tend to estimate the expected length of stay and initiate plans to ensure that social care, community nursing or GP support and equipment are available when needed and do not delay the discharge if the patient is well enough to return home.

There are examples from across the country of discharge processes that are better than some others – perhaps where personal care contracts are maintained for up to seventy-two hours after a person is admitted to hospital, allowing for them to be stabilised or treated and returned home without delay, knowing that their usual carers will be there to settle them in and make sure they have everything they need. Or maybe working with a local voluntary organisation to provide home-from-hospital befriending support, where the discharged patient has a visitor to make sure they have all they need in the first few days or weeks after discharge. It could be providing milk and bread boxes – a local supermarket donating goods to provide sufficient supplies for someone to eat and drink for a few days.

There are always likely to be challenges associated with discharge processes due to assessment delays, care package delays or family members not agreeing on placement delays. However, NHS Trust leaders need to understand why delays are occurring and what measures would be most effective in supporting people to get home. This should involve both inward-monitoring and review, and review, and an outward-facing system giving consideration to possible solutions. It can be difficult to step aside from the usual solutions to persistent problems and to see new potential solutions, but clinging to actions that don't work well is in nobody's best interests. Often it needs a multi-pronged approach, but with clear oversight and accountability.

---

83 Rojas-García A, Turner S, Pizzo E, et al (2018) Impact and experiences of delayed discharge: a mixed-studies systematic review. Health Expect 21: 41–56.

84 Lack of social care has led to 2.5 million lost bed days in the NHS between the last Election and this one. Age UK 2019.

An example – Emily

Building on good practice is always the best way to drive improvements, but the following story takes a little while to get to a good ending – all because transition planning was pushed down the priority list. It is an entirely true story.

A seventeen-year-old girl – let's call her Emily – falls from a horse and sustains life-changing injuries, including a serious head injury. She is airlifted to a tertiary centre that offers paediatric neurosurgery and critical care facilities. It is a teaching hospital with a medical school at the nearby Russell Group university. Emily has surgery and is in the paediatric critical care unit for about nine weeks. Her parents are told to prepare for the worst, but Emily survives. After another few weeks on the children's ward, she is transferred to the paediatric assessment and rehabilitation centre where she is offered a comprehensive programme of activities, therapy, education and psychological support. Her parents visit every day and are welcomed as an integral part of the team.

Emily slowly learns to walk and talk again. There are anomalies that help her parents and staff to realise there is hope for the future – for instance, Emily has not lost the ability to tie shoelaces despite initially not being able to put her shoes on herself. She knows the words but can't say them in the right order, so she speaks in a stream of unconnected words. She knows that this is happening, and she becomes frustrated with herself when her ability to put words in the correct order is used to explain how she is feeling. "Oh, for (expletive's) sake, stupid (another expletive) words!"

Everyone is delighted that Emily is alive and making steady progress. They know that it is a long-haul fix, and that some parts of Emily will be changed forever. The service from the Trust is exemplary… until about a month before Emily reaches her eighteenth birthday, when her parents receive a note saying simply that, as Emily will become an adult, she will no longer be allowed to remain on the paediatric rehabilitation unit and her parents must find alternative provision.

They have no idea where to start. The nurse specialist is unhelpful, telling them that no discussion is needed as there are two funded places that would probably accept Emily. The nurse suggests they visit. One is a care home specialising in care for people with acquired or progressive neurological impairment. Most of the people living there are over sixty years old, have long-term effects of strokes or are in the final stages of degenerative conditions such as Huntingdon's disease. It is a nice enough home, but entirely unsuitable for the intensive rehabilitation and forward planning that Emily needs. Bizarrely, it agrees to take her, but Emily's parents are not in agreement, particularly as they have seen someone with obvious disinhibited behaviour and feel that

Emily is young and vulnerable. They visit the second service, where they are told that Emily will only be allowed visitors at the weekend and 'home leave' is just once a month as she needs to settle and learn independence. Her parents want her to go back to school, to have a future, and not to live forever in an institution that fails to see their daughter as a person.

The Trust staff are still remarkably unhelpful, saying they need the bed for a child and it is unsuitable for an adult so Emily must leave. They refuse to engage until the words, "Unsafe Discharge, Children Act (1989)", "safeguarding", and "Education, Health and Care plan" are mentioned.[85] Emily's parents then ask to meet with the lead paediatrician, the CEO of the Trust, a hospital social worker and someone from the Clinical Commissioning Group (as was), and explain that they have a plan and that this is in Emily's best interests. They ask that Emily be discharged to their care – reminding them that, as Emily is over sixteen years of age and they have no Lasting Power of Attorney, it has to be a best interest decision. Discharging her to an entirely inappropriate setting is not in her best interest.

They identify providers of physiotherapy and speech therapy near the family home, ask for a support worker to give Emily some independence and help her engage in the community, and ask the Trust to work with the local authority to provide an EHCP to enable Emily to continue to study and have her needs properly assessed – and reassessed as they change over time. There is some pushback because this isn't the norm (although life-changing injuries from a riding accident aren't the norm, either). The parents then play their trump card, which is that, for all the agencies involved, it is cheaper if they work together to facilitate the plan that the parents have suggested. Emily's father is an accountant, and he understands that money talks.

Emily is given a six-week discharge package of support, and then has to reapply (why do we make it so difficult when life is hard enough for some people?). She eventually secures the funding to pay for the support she needs to sustain her recovery and maximise her potential. She returns to school to repeat the sixth form year (with an assistant and enhanced IT equipment), and she gets a job in a small garden centre for three hours on Saturdays. Today, Emily is working on a supported summer internship which will hopefully boost her confidence, her independence, and help prepare her for university. She has a place on a foundation degree course in October; she is really excited about it, although her parents are terrified!

How much better if the hospital that saved Emily's life, and provided very good care when she was critically ill and recovering, had also thought about her upcoming transition, and had helped her and her parents to plan rather than battling them?

---

85   See www.gov.uk/children-with-special-educational-needs/extra-SEN-help (accessed August 2023).

Planning for transitions

This Quality Statement is not just about acute hospitals; it applies wherever people move between services either permanently or on a temporary basis.

Adult social care providers need to think about how best to support people who require hospital admission and how to ensure that, for those unable to communicate their own needs, that there are systems or processes to ensure that essential information is passed over. 'I am me' style passports that detail people's preferences and other information are only useful if they are current, completed, and travel with the person. Providers may want to think about whether it is appropriate and safe to send someone off in an ambulance or to an appointment using hospital transport without someone familiar, who knows them well, to support them.

Ambulance providers will want to think about what information they need to have when they collect someone to transfer from home or an adult social care setting to a hospital or vice versa. That might be checking that the person has their hearing aids, their glasses, a phone, their 'I am me' passport or other essentials that could be missed. They certainly need contact details of the home or a person to call. Having those things smooths transitions. Ambulance providers supporting people in need of a secure environment need to ensure that they have the necessary information about potential triggers that might result in violence or self-harm and the legal status of the person, so they know what the limits of their remit are. Of course, the provider of the service the person is coming from should offer it, but the accepting ambulance is also responsible for ensuring they have the correct information to meet people's needs.

Children's hospices and children's hospitals need to consider adulthood. Just like Emily, many of the children they support will eventually need to move across to adult services. There needs to be a clear policy around that. When children's hospices started up across the country, there was not always full consideration of this, and there were often applications to vary admission criteria so that a child reaching adulthood could still be cared for in a familiar environment that they and their parents knew. It didn't help that there was so little respite and support for a seriously unwell or disabled young adult, and that as a result parents often applied pressure, not unreasonably, to have their child remain on the books.

Some hospices decided to build units or separate young-adult facilities. Opened in 2004, Douglas House was linked to Helen House, the first children's hospice in the UK. It cared for young adults aged between sixteen and thirty-five as the world's first specialist hospice exclusively for young adults that bridged the gap between a children's and adult's hospice. Douglas House closed on 21st June 2018 due to a shortfall in funding, but Helen House remains open to care for terminally ill babies, children and young people up to the age of eighteen.

Similarly, Jack's Place in Winchester continues to provide care for young adults who have 'moved up' from Naomi House, the sister children's hospice.[86] The provider had thought about transition, and how the needs of young adults were different to the needs of children, and planned to ensure that the transition was as smooth as possible. Other children's hospices have adapted their Statement of Purpose, and have made plans for individual children either to transfer or to continue to be supported by the children's hospices – knowing that their prognosis is very poor, that their lives are likely to be short and that the support they are offered enables them to continue to live in ways that are as fulfilling as possible as their bodies fail them.

Children's hospitals and services caring for children with long-term conditions need to be able to demonstrate that they have planned for adulthood, and that they have thought about what a young person wants and what is in their best interests. Conversely, adult services accepting young adults need to plan for the transition from the opposite direction. Services for young adults with learning disabilities, autism or mental health conditions need to be able to demonstrate that they think about the changes the young person faces and plan care accordingly. That might be with independence plans and a gradual increase in freedoms, it might involve helping with access to contraception, or might be about encouraging self-determination. It is a transition, and it needs recognition and planning for.

The final transition, of course, is when life ends (although some will believe that there are more transitions after bodily death, and that needs respecting). People may move between services quite rapidly and, given that we each die only once, there is only one opportunity to get it right. There really should be a seamless transition, with carefully planned and communicated arrangements that might negate the need for moving between services.

Hospitals, hospices, community healthcare services, the voluntary sector (Marie Curie nurses, for example), ambulance services, social care settings and GPs all need to plan for this inevitable eventuality. It is not helpful if a GP signs a 'Do Not Attempt Cardio-Pulmonary Resuscitation' (DNACPR) form correctly and appropriately, but the home files it away and calls an ambulance when someone who is already actively dying develops a changed breathing pattern. The ambulance crew might ask about DNACPR, get a blank look from the agency nurse on duty, and so transport the patient to hospital where they sit for two hours before their heart stops. Or perhaps nobody has thought about completing a DNACPR form, so the junior doctor presses the alarm, starts vigorous cardiac massage and continues until the consultant arrives and tells them to stop. That isn't nice for anyone involved, and certainly not for the deceased person or their family.

---

86 www.naomihouse.org.uk/about-us/jacksplace (accessed August 2023).

Proper planning for these transfers between providers is an essential of good care delivery. That includes when there is a need for people to transfer between services in an emergency, which means independent healthcare services having processes in place to support urgent transfers when someone's condition deteriorates, or if the independent service cannot provide the care needed. Perhaps a probable cancer is diagnosed during an MRI scan, but there are no cancer treatment facilities – staff need to know how to ensure that the diagnosis is followed up, and not left in an email to a consultant that no longer works at the local Trust.

Protected characteristics and specific needs

As with most aspects of care and treatment, it is service dependent, and providers need to think about the transitions faced by the people they work with. There has to be consideration of people from specific groups who have protected characteristics, and how their transitions will be managed so that the risks associated with moving between providers are reduced. Groups where careful consideration of how their needs can be met is required to avoid them falling between gaps in services include:

- Gypsy, Roma and Traveller people who may move around the country and miss out on vital services, and who also have difficulty accessing services when they are settled. That should be a consideration for school nurses, midwifery services, health visitors, GP practices, children's hospices, palliative care teams and many others.

- Children and adults with complex care needs, particularly those placed a long distance from their families. This includes people with learning disabilities, physical disabilities, mental health conditions, autism and long-term or life limiting conditions. Most parents of children and young people with disabilities will talk at length about battling to get their child the care and treatment they need. Some can't even get assessed, so they don't have a formal diagnosis and can't claim benefits. If you support someone who may need hearing aids, glasses, walking aids, complex medication, respite care, incontinence support, speech and language support, physiotherapy and surgery to manage spinal deformities or contractures, and those services are all contracted out to different providers, life becomes one long round of making and attending appointments.

- People living with dementia who may still be at home with a spouse, but with increasing needs. There may well be numerous transitions to hospital, to community hospital, to adult social care settings and possibly an 'in-house' transition where there is a need to support the person to accept community health and domiciliary care. The unfamiliar can be very distressing, and what appears to be disease progression may simply be a reaction to changes.

- People with sensory loss. Accessing services can be a challenge at the best of times, but for people with sensory loss it can be really frustrating. Lack of communication and lack of planning for transitions may leave people unable to interpret their environment or communicate their preferences and needs. They may fall down gaps between services because they don't know the gaps are there.

- People who are very obese and require specialist bariatric support alongside their other care needs. Discharging bigger patients from hospital, either to their own home or to a care home, can be challenging. Many do not have the resources, the staffing and the equipment. A third of respondents in a US study reported being unable to transfer these patients, sometimes with delays of weeks or even months.[87] This is likely to be a more frequent challenge with a recent study noting increases in enquiries about possible admittance to care homes by people with extreme obesity (BMI ≥40) who may require bariatric equipment.[88] This group will use most types of setting, and the movement between services can often be fraught with difficulties.

Evidence to support the Quality Statement

What evidence can you have to support the claim that you are meeting the required standards for this Quality Statement? The two most important areas will be around policy – having a clear service policy around transitions, and ensuring that it is followed – and feedback from those who have used the service and have actually experienced its approach to transitions in practice.

Evidence from data and records

The obvious starting point is having policies that address transition. In the case of childhood to adulthood, that might be a transition policy. A care home for older people might want a hospital admission policy, and an ambulance provider might want a protocol around collecting people from a care home. A community service working with Gypsy, Roma and Traveller people might want a service map that helps staff and the people using the service to understand what services are available and how to access them; it would be better, perhaps, as a system-wide map, but staff who work directly with people needing to access services might find it useful.

---

87   Bradway CK, Felix HC, Whitfield T (2017) Barriers in transitioning patients with severe obesity from hospitals to nursing homes. *West J Nurs Res* **39** (3) 1151–1168.

88   Thompson J (2021) An exploration of the challenges of providing person-centred care for older care home residents with obesity. *Health and Social Care* **30** (4) e1112–e1122.

The caveat around communication with other providers and shared care is around consent. While it is good practice to keep involved agencies and other providers informed, people using the service have a right to privacy and consent is needed before sharing information and discharging someone to the care of another provider. Not every woman will want her GP to know that she has had a termination of pregnancy, and that is her right – even if the advice is that the doctor performing surgery noticed a lump that they felt needed investigating.

The policy or policies need to be known. In acute independent healthcare hospitals, the resident medical officer usually changes quite frequently. As the on-site doctor, they need to know when and how to transfer someone to the local NHS hospital for emergency care, and they probably won't have time to look at the policy on the computer when someone is septic.

The policy needs to be implemented, and people's records need to show the discussions, consents, arrangements and timeline for a move that is planned. Ideally the planning should take place over a period of time that allows for changes and for alternatives, if necessary. Children don't suddenly become adults; well, strictly speaking they do become adults on their eighteenth birthday, but that doesn't come as a surprise! It is known well in advance that adulthood is approaching, and the preparation should begin some years ahead of any move, if possible.

In the same way, for many patients, there can be an estimated discharge date, and the planning towards that can commence well ahead of time so as to avoid delays caused by a lack of a care package, or worse, the person being sent home without any care having been arranged. If someone is likely to be moving into or returning to residential care following a spell in hospital, the care home provider needs to make an assessment and ensure that they can meet or continue to meet that person's needs. Specialist equipment may be needed, and that takes time, but isn't usually a surprise on the day of discharge; people who are likely to need a pressure-relieving mattress usually have that need identified during their stay, and so plans can be made to have one provided at the care home. Timeliness is good when planning for transition, and it often saves work later on.

Transitions need to be monitored. Almost every hospital in the country will have complaints and incidents about unsafe discharges, often compounded by a lack of communication. This is sometimes accepted as the norm, and it shouldn't be. It's a failing and one that may have a higher profile in inspection reports now there is a Quality Statement specifically around transitions. What does monitoring look like? There can be data sets around expected and delayed discharges, capacity, and length of stay. There can be data around time from prescribing drugs to take home (TTOs) to the drugs being provided. Hopefully, planning will mean TTOs were ordered a day or even two days before the patient was discharged, particularly if the discharge is planned for a weekend.

Evidence from staff and service users

For this Quality Statement, the best evidence is that provided by people who have used the service and who have moved from one setting to another. Asking people for feedback is a good way, although it has to be specific and you have to ask the right questions. When that is the case, it will sometimes reveal unexpected root causes.

Focus groups and patient participation groups can help providers such as hospitals and GPs to understand the gaps. The local Healthwatch might be persuaded to carry out a project around discharges. A phone call to people who have moved from a service might be useful feedback, and people will usually appreciate the provider asking. Not all NHS hospital patients can be asked by telephone – that would be impractical – but someone from the Patient Advice and Liaison Service (PALS) or a student nurse, with a project to write up, might be able to call care homes where people have been discharged to and ask the manager about any problems. Community hospital providers could do the same, as there tend to be fewer people being discharged at any one time. Most independent acute hospitals could (and sometimes do) call patients who have been discharged. They could include specific questions about transitions and the co-ordination of care with other providers.

How providers choose to ask people using their service is ultimately up to them; the important thing is that they do ask.

If there is an issue identified around transitions, and particularly if there is a pattern identified, then the problem needs to be understood and addressed. There needs to be evidence that any action plans are both implemented and effective. If 'reminding ward doctors to prescribe TTOs before 9am' is not working because the doctors have a ward round then, all the reminders in the world, in flashing lights and glitter fountains won't improve the situation. Change the process instead!

Monitoring emergency transitions is harder. It would be inappropriate to phone the spouse of a patient who had died in an ambulance on the way to an emergency department to ask how the move went. To offer condolences, perhaps, but not for details of the move. It might be better, as part of the emergency transfer policy, to have a debrief session included as standard for all those involved. The session could be a standard agenda that included whether policy was followed and any problems around that. That provides evidence, and also identifies whether a policy is followed in practice.

If the monitoring shows that transitions work well, that's very good. Note the review date on the policy and keep it as it is for the time being. If there are challenges, consult and understand what needs changing, and then change the policy and add a new review date, which allows for further monitoring.

Chapter 13: Safeguarding

Quality Statement:

We work with people to understand what being safe means to them as well as with our partners on the best way to achieve this. We concentrate on improving people's lives while protecting their right to live in safety, free from bullying, harassment, abuse, discrimination, avoidable harm and neglect. We make sure we share concerns quickly and appropriately.

All providers should be able to say without hesitation that they meet this standard. Sadly, they can't always do so, or at least they can't evidence that they do so. It is about far more than completing mandatory training and having a safeguarding policy that is current. They are essential, of course, but they are not enough to make a service stand out as particularly good or better.

In considering this Quality Statement, it is useful to identify which regulations it maps to. As already explained it is regulations, not Quality Statements, that are breached. The main regulations suggested by the Commission as linked to this statement are:

- Regulation 11: 'Need for consent'.
- Regulation 12: 'Safe care and treatment'.
- Regulation 13: 'Safeguarding service users from abuse and improper treatment'.

There are also other linked regulations which might be breached if this Quality Statement is not fully met. These include Regulation 9: 'Person-centred care', Regulation 17: 'Good governance' and Regulation 20: 'Duty of candour'.

The first part of this Quality Statement is an interesting addition to the regulatory framework: "We work with people to understand what being safe means to them". It links to the need to obtain consent and to the Mental Capacity Act (2005), and particularly to the Mental Capacity Act Deprivation of Liberty Safeguards (DoLS). Many providers will also need to consider the Mental Health Act (2007), which is a law used in England and Wales to provide a legal framework for both informal and compulsory care and treatment of people diagnosed with having a mental disorder. This applies not only to specialist psychiatric services, but also to acute hospitals, general practice, urgent treatment centres and many ambulance services.

Staff in health and social care services are usually nice, kind people. They want the best for those they work with – they want to keep them safe, to help them get better if they are ill, and to prevent them hurting themselves.

That can be the exact opposite of upholding people's right to choose and to make unwise decisions when they have the capacity to do so. Even where people lack capacity for a specific decision (and capacity is always decision-specific), the person is entitled to minimal restrictions on their liberty and maximum support to make their own decisions. That doesn't just mean whether they want sugar in their tea or whether to wear their blue or green shirt. It means being involved in every decision that affects them. It means letting them take risks when they choose and have capacity to do so. That can sit very uncomfortably with many care providers. It also means, for many healthcare professionals, that assessing capacity accurately is complex and, in many cases, requires expert input.

Providers need to be able to evidence that not only have they followed the principles of the Mental Capacity Act (2005) and have policies and guidance in place for staff, but that they seek expert advice and input where it is hard to decide whether someone has capacity for a specific decision. Living in a care home does not mean you have to sit in a communal lounge watching daytime television or joining in the weekly singalong if you want to do something else. It doesn't mean you have to eat with others if you prefer to eat alone. It doesn't mean you have to have a weekly bath, or that you cannot have a daily bath if you want one. If we're being honest, routines and restrictions are usually there to benefit the staff and make them feel more comfortable, rather than for the benefit of residents or patients.

Two examples – freedom of choice

Two examples come to mind. One involves a care home in which a small group of men wrote on the 'wishing tree' that they wanted to go to a gentleman's club to watch 'dancing' (my euphemism not theirs.) Instead of laughing and telling the men they were too old, or ignoring the request, the care home staff arranged a visit to a strip club and the men enjoyed a beer while watching a table dance. Whatever you think of the sex-work industry, the men were supported to make their own choices. The same home also acknowledged a resident's choice to remain sexually active; they facilitated contact with a sex worker who visited the home regularly and met in private with the resident. Very few people knew about this; it wasn't considered a bigger risk than other visitors (usually family and friends) having time in private with other residents. The same security arrangements were followed for all visitors, and the same courtesy was extended to all. There was no discernible difference in the way the visiting sex worker was treated to the way a visiting church minister was treated, and that lack of judgement allowed the man to live his life as he chose.

The second example came from a recent social media exchange around people living in care homes and very warm weather. A member of staff from a care home was saying they had a difficult situation where a couple of 'their' residents refused to stay in the shade and refused suncream. They were so bold as to suggest they liked a suntan and the warmth of a summer day on their skin. One even took his shirt off and stayed outside in the midday sun. There was significant debate about whether to allow them outside if they had suncream on first or to insist they came in for drinks and lunch. One staff member even suggested locking external doors. There was very little consideration that these people had been enjoying the sun for the best part of eighty years, had the capacity to continue to enjoy the sun, and had the right to get burned if they wanted. Given that Vitamin D deficiency is widespread and severe in elderly men, especially those living in institutions, and many dieticians suggest that Vitamin D supplementation should be routinely prescribed in institutions for the elderly, the residents sunbathing might be no bad thing.[89] That said, the point is not whether sunbathing is beneficial or harmful, it's about staff thinking they have a right, or indeed a responsibility, to make 'wise' decisions for people they are supporting.

Capacity and consent

Even worse than a belief among staff that they must make decisions for the people they care for is the blanket assumption that anyone over about sixty-five might not have capacity. The law requires an assumption of capacity, yet so often that is ignored. I have seen reports of independent hospitals where a capacity assessment of all patients admitted for surgery was presented as a positive finding; it isn't, it is bordering on abusive and certainly discriminatory on grounds of age. Older people usually have capacity, and those that don't may have fluctuating capacity and so should be offered the chance to make a decision at the time when they are most able to make it.

Similarly, consent by children is often only partially followed. The guidance has changed, and the laws have different applicable ages, which further complicates matters. The guiding principle is always that providers and healthcare professionals must act in the best interests of the children they are treating. Deciding what is in their best interests is not always easy, and paragraph 24 of the General Medical Council guidance merits further consideration.[90] It states, "You must decide whether a young person is able to understand the nature, purpose and possible consequences of investigations or treatments you propose, as well as the consequences of not having treatment. Only if they are able to understand, retain, use and weigh this information, and communicate their decision to others, can they consent to that investigation or treatment."

---

89 Boüüaert C, Vanmeerbeek M, Burette P, *et al* (2008) Vitamin D deficiency in elderly men living in urban areas, at home or in institutions. *Presse Medicale* **37** (2 part 1) 191 – 200

90 www.gmc-uk.org/ethical-guidance/ethical-guidance-for-doctors/0-18-years/making-decisions (accessed August 2023.

This is the opposite of the Mental Capacity Act (2005) principles that say you must assume capacity, unless there is reason to think there may be a lack of capacity. Children over sixteen are covered by the Mental Capacity Act, and healthcare services assume that they are competent to give consent for any treatment, unless there is another reason to consider they may lack capacity (such as a learning disability or significant mental health concerns). Providers and staff providing care and treatment for children under sixteen must be able to demonstrate that they have assessed the ability of the child to understand the nature, purpose and possible consequences of proposed investigations or treatments, as well as the consequences of not having treatment. That requires staff to make an assessment, and to record why they believe a child is competent to understand what is being suggested and to weigh up the benefits and risks. Simply having a child turn up on their own is not enough. If a child cannot be shown to be able to assimilate and process the information about the procedure, then the guidance requires that parental consent is sought.

The consent guidance from the General Medical Council is in line with the Frazer Guidelines which specifically relate only to contraception and sexual health (and are not the same as Gillick Competence). They are named after one of the Lords who was responsible for the Gillick judgement, but who went on to address the specific issue of giving contraceptive advice and treatment to under sixteens without parental consent. The guidance allows for advice and treatment to be given in this situation as long as:

- The child has sufficient maturity and intelligence to understand the nature and implications of the proposed treatment.
- The child cannot be persuaded to tell his or her parents or to allow the doctor to tell them.
- The child is very likely to begin or continue having sexual intercourse with or without contraceptive treatment.
- The child's physical or mental health is likely to suffer unless he or she receives the advice or treatment.
- The advice or treatment is in the young person's best interests.

The guidance is that health professionals should still encourage the young person to inform his or her parent(s) or get permission to do so on their behalf, but if this permission is not given they can still give the child advice and treatment assuming the other conditions are met.

Safeguarding and discrimination

Consent is a safeguarding issue, but the two are often not connected in the minds of staff. In the sunbathing scenario, the staff posting comments on Twitter undoubtedly felt that by preventing the carcinogenic effects of sunshine and possible sunburn on elderly residents, they were protecting them from harm – and thus safeguarding them. In fact, the very opposite is true. They were trying to unlawfully restrict people's freedom. Sunbathing may not seem a particularly important decision one way or the other. If stopped from going outside in the midday sun, most people would find something else to do and shrug when required to eat their lunch indoors. Imagine, then, if the staff then protected people in more intrusive ways – for instance deciding that their relationship with another resident was unhealthy and moving one of them to another home, or deciding that someone might fall if they tried walking around unaided and so taking their walking frame away from them, or allowing a daughter to visit even if the resident said they didn't want them allowed in. Without consent laws and guidance being used appropriately and recorded as such, people are not being protected from harm and abuse and are not being supported to live their life as they want.

Discrimination is also mentioned, and it may feel to some as if that shouldn't necessarily sit alongside safeguarding. Most people would say racism was wrong, but they might not see it as connected to protecting people from harm in most situations. Until, that is, they consider the harms caused to certain groups because they have a protected characteristic. Equality and diversity are threads that should run through all areas of practice and employment. If this doesn't happen, then the service is likely to be failing to protect many people. All policies should consider the impact on people using the service and staff with protected characteristics. Every inspection should consider the outcomes of specific groups, too – but that is a work in progress, and the good provider can be a bit ahead of the field by providing evidence that they do consider this as part of their governance.

There is increasing recognition that there are many avoidable deaths of people with learning disabilities. The rates of premature and 'amenable' deaths are substantially higher for people with learning disabilities than for those in the general population. Research data shows that 28% of deaths reported were 'amenable' – in other words, that current knowledge suggests that most or all deaths from that cause could have been avoided through the provision of good quality healthcare.[91] Almost half (42%) of the 244 deaths reviewed showed that they were premature, in that specific adverse events were identified in the pathway leading to death that, if prevented, would probably have allowed the person to live for at least another year. The English Learning Disabilities Mortality Review (LeDeR) programme shows some progress in addressing the care deficits for people with learning disabilities, but there is more to do.

---

91   Heslop P *et al* (2013) *Confidential Inquiry into Premature Deaths of People with Learning Disabilities* [online]. Norah Fry Research Centre: Bristol. Available at: www.bristol.ac.uk/media-library/sites/cipold/migrated/documents/fullfinalreport.pdf (accessed August 2023).

It would be easy to think that this was a problem specifically related to acute hospital care, but of course that is not true. The healthcare of people with learning disabilities is usually the responsibility of many providers, and all have a shared responsibility to ensure equity of access and equity of outcomes. That means care home providers and supported-living providers advocating for the people they support, and identifying and responding to concerns.

A report published by NICE showed the disparity of access for women with a learning disability to breast cancer screening.[92] The proportion of women aged fifty to sixty-nine with a learning disability who received breast cancer screening was 51%. This compares to 65% of women in the same age group without a learning disability. If breast cancer is diagnosed at an early stage, it is often curable and certainly treatable. If women are not offered screening, diagnosis may only be made at a much later stage. Adult social care providers need to ensure they have guidance for staff about healthcare needs and to advocate for women to support them to access mammography services, if they wish.

GP practices should also have annual health checks in place for people with learning disabilities.[93] Evidence suggests that providing health checks to people with learning disabilities in primary care is effective in identifying previously unrecognised health needs, including those associated with life-threatening illnesses. NHS England have set a target that 75% of eligible people will have an annual health check by 2023/24. Their website gives examples of where this happening, and how the local systems are making it work.[94] It would be hard for a GP practice to argue that they were 'Outstanding' if they had not delivered annual health checks for the majority of their patients with a learning disability.

We know that black babies are more likely to be stillborn, or to die in the perinatal period.[95] We also know that infant death can be linked to poverty, and that the perinatal mortality rates are higher in areas of greatest socio-economic challenge. There are undoubtedly many factors that affect these tragic outcomes, but not all are about lifestyle choices or genetics. Research in the US showed that the perinatal mortality rate for black

92 NICE (2021) *NICE impact people with a learning disability* [online]. Available at: www.nice.org. uk/about/what-we-do/into-practice/measuring-the-use-of-nice-guidance/impact-of-our-guidance/ nice-impact-people-with-a-learning-disability (accessed August 2023).

93 PHE (2016) *Annual health checks and people with learning disabilities* [online]. Available at: www.gov.uk/government/publications/annual-health-checks-and-people-with-learning-disabilities/ annual-health-checks-and-people-with-learning-disabilities (accessed August 2023).

94 www.england.nhs.uk/learning-disabilities/improving-health/annual-health-checks/ (accessed August 2023).

95 ONS (2022) Child and infant mortality in England and Wales: 2020 [online]. Available at: www.ons.gov.uk/peoplepopulationandcommunity/birthsdeathsandmarriages/deaths/bulletins/ childhoodinfantandperinatalmortalityinenglandandwales/2020 (accessed August 2023).

babies fell when the mothers were cared for by black doctors.[96] That rather suggests that some baby deaths are avoidable deaths.

Is discrimination a safeguarding issue? I would argue that, if people died because of a protected characteristic, it is a very serious safeguarding issue. Preventable harm doesn't get much worse than avoidable death. I think this raises questions about whether it is a national issue, something that needs the national agencies to work together to address, or something that providers can begin to address themselves. My view, and the view of the Commission, is that discrimination is something that everyone should be concerned about, and something that all providers should want to consider when reviewing their policies, training and governance processes.

An example – learning disability and discrimination

A situation was shared with me in which a forty-three-year-old woman with a learning disability was admitted with an obstructed bowel and gravely ill from aspiration pneumonia. The admitting surgeon's view was that it was inappropriate to treat her in critical care as her quality of life was so limited and the obstruction was probably a malignancy, and likely to be quite advanced. They sought palliative medicine input about symptom control, but the palliative care consultant pointed out that the conversation would not be happening if the patient did not have a learning disability. The argument about quality of life came up again, with the surgeon failing to fully grasp that it was not for him to judge the value of someone else's life.

The woman was transferred to critical care and her family visited. She had been out to lunch with her young nieces when she aspirated something while laughing. Her nieces were very fond of their aunt who brought them presents, did colouring with them and paddled in the sea with them. Not a life without value, by anyone's standards. There might be an argument (which was mooted at the time) that this was likely to be an advanced malignancy, and it was unfair to put someone through a brutal treatment regime when they had a learning disability. That misses the point completely: the woman had a reversible aspiration pneumonia, she was entitled to the same care as everyone else and the conversation about critical care would not have taken place had she not had a learning disability.

In this case, the issue was the staff making decisions beyond their remit and deciding on someone's quality of life without really exploring what that life was like. It is for providers to support staff through training, supervision and a learning culture to ensure that care and treatment is delivered without prejudice. Unequal care is unsafe care.

---

96 Mahase E (2020) Black babies are less likely to die when cared for by black doctors, US study finds. *BMJ* 370.

Best interest decisions

The example above brings us to the idea of best interest decisions. I have no doubt the surgeon thought he was making a best interest decision. As the woman was so unwell, a Do Not Attempt Cardio-Pulmonary Resuscitation decision might well have been appropriate on grounds of futility – but that should be done in consultation with the family. NICE has a quality standard [QS194] 'Decision-making and mental capacity' which says, "People aged sixteen and over who lack capacity to make a particular decision at the time that decision needs to be made have their wishes, feelings, values and beliefs accounted for in best interests decisions."[97] The surgeon above did not take those wishes, feelings, values and beliefs into account when deciding that palliative care was more appropriate than active management of a reversible condition. He didn't know the woman's family would want to take her home and, when the time came, to support her to have a comfortable death surrounded by people that loved her. It is possible that appropriate treatment may well have allowed the woman more several years of life. He hadn't seen the person, just a learning disability.

NICE says that:

"The person must be placed at the heart of the decision-making process and supported to be involved in the decision-making process as far as possible. Wherever possible this means finding out about the person's past and present wishes, feelings, values and beliefs that would have influenced the decision if the person had capacity. It also means using information included in care plans and advance care plans, consulting with the person's family, carers and advocates and seeking to establish the person's wishes, preferences, and values."

Does this happen in your organisation?

NICE goes on to suggest that: "For adults (aged eighteen and over), particular attention should be paid to advance decisions, Lasting Power of Attorney and court order, including any court-appointed deputy." I know that all-too-often services accept that when a person says they are 'next-of-kin' that is accepted as spoken, when the term 'next-of-kin' has no legal status when it comes to decision-making. It is far easier to consult the people standing beside someone's bed than to ask to see the documents that give them decision-making rights, but that doesn't mean that the person who happened to be the first to pop in and find someone semi-conscious after a stroke is necessarily the legal representative or the only person who should be consulted. All services where best interest decisions are made need to ensure that they have a process for checking the status

---

97 https://www.nice.org.uk/guidance/qs194/chapter/Quality-statement-4-Best-interests-decision-making Accessed 14.6.2023

of the people claiming decision-making rights. Sadly, money matters are occasionally at the forefront of some relatives' minds, and decisions are made at their behest which are about preserving assets rather than doing what is actually in the person's best interests.

NICE recommends that providers offer their staff a toolkit to support them in carrying out and recording best interest decisions. The legal requirement is more complex than a consultant, GP, social worker, nurse, paramedic or other professional simply thinking that something is best for the person before them. The toolkit (which should form part of the policy) should include details such as:

■ Identifying any decision-making instruments that would have an impact on best interests decision-making (a registered Lasting Power of Attorney, a deputy, advance decisions to refuse treatment, court orders).

■ When to seek the support of an Independent Mental Capacity Advocate and how to do this.

■ A reminder to consult those who should be consulted such as all close family members and spouses, friends (possibly), partners, advocates and relevant professionals.

■ Guidance about how and where to record the best interest decision. NICE suggests a template that offers a balance sheet to enable all information to be considered, and which forms a record of the risks and benefits.

■ Guidance about what information to record and where. This must cover a clear explanation of the decision to be made and what support a person has had to enable them to make their own decision. It should include a current assessment that shows the person lacks capacity to make the decision being discussed and a record of their wishes and preferences (if known or ascertainable).

■ The record should include the choices the person has been offered and the important information they would need to understand to make that decision.

■ Then there should be a signed record of the best interest decision, with the reasons and names and roles of those making the decision.

Evidence to support the Quality Statement

As with most Quality Statements, documents and data are the easiest form of evidence to provide to an inspection team, or to supply via the portal to reduce the risk rating that the Commission has for the service. Evidence from staff and people using the service will then follow on from the documentary evidence.

Evidence from data and records

There need to be policies aligned to best-practice guidelines and the legislative frameworks. These need to be current, regularly reviewed, and accessible and known to staff. Which policies there are and what they cover will be service-specific, but most will require a consent policy, a safeguarding policy and a responding to allegations policy (that may form part of the safeguarding policy) as a minimum. There might also be a need for a restraint policy, and a separate policy or section of a policy about the Mental Health Act and how it impacts on the service provided.

A care home for older people will need a consent policy that covers the Mental Capacity Act (2005) and which also guides staff about the remit and limits of a Lasting Power of Attorney – but which is not likely to need a section on consent by children under sixteen years of age. A GP practice will need a consent policy that covers all ages, as well as the mental capacity and mental health legislation. A private ambulance provider will need to think about their statement of purpose and who they provide care or treatment to when they write their consent policy. Most providers' consent policies will need to cover the Lasting Power of Attorney's role and ensure that those who claim to hold delegated powers do actually hold them. There needs to be a section on who can make best interest decisions when this is appropriate, and who should be consulted.

Acceptable behaviours are something we hope we all demonstrate and recognise, and which we expect all staff to know and show at all times. This doesn't always happen, sadly. Human factors come into play, with overstretched, tired and stressed staff tending to be snappier and less tolerant. It's not all about human factors though. The Royal College of Surgeons published a guidance document called *Managing Disruptive Behaviours in Surgery – A guide to good practice* in 2021.[98] Similarly, the Joint Commission in the US issued a Sentinel Event Alert in 2008, citing evidence that intimidating and disruptive behaviours can, among other things, "foster

---

98 www.rcseng.ac.uk/standards-and-research/standards-and-guidance/good-practice-guides/managing-disruptive-behaviours/ (accessed August 2023).

medical errors" and contribute to "preventable adverse outcomes", and should not be tolerated.[99]

The US isn't alone in having unreasonable behaviours that affect the way care and treatment is delivered: bad behaviour is a safety issue. In 2019, *The British Medical Journal* reported that a review by the Royal College of Surgeons had found that, in over half of the surgical reviews, there were concerns about the inappropriate behaviour of a surgeon or about a lack of respect between surgeons and within teams. The report said that surgeons in difficulty could become dismissive when concerns were raised about their behaviour, and could become "difficult to manage, controlling, or arrogant in their approach."[100]

It's not only surgeons, of course, and not only in acute hospitals where we see poor behaviour impacting on outcomes for people using services. One only has to look back to the Winterbourne View case to see that all services can witness very inappropriate behaviour towards people using services or other staff. Providers need to ensure their systems and monitoring processes identify and address these behaviours with a zero-tolerance approach to bullying, harassment and sexually inappropriate or aggressive behaviours towards others using or working at the service.

An example – culture change

How can one change the culture of a setting or a service? It's not easy, and it takes a while for new behaviours to embed, generally. Part of it is in the messaging that is received by other staff. One newly appointed CEO, who took over the leadership of a Trust rated 'Inadequate' and placed in special measures, told the inspection team he was going to see the Trust become 'Outstanding' before he retired. The culture of the Trust was its major downfall, with demoralised staff, leaders who were dismissive of patient safety concerns, a 'them and us' culture at its worst in the operating theatres and an unwillingness of senior leaders to see what was happening.

The CEO spent his first few days walking around speaking to staff in all areas of the hospital. He sent his executive team out to do likewise, and one spent some time observing in the operating department and on the surgical wards. It was obvious that one very senior surgeon was behaving appallingly - throwing things around the theatre and ward, shouting at nurses and junior doctors, snapping at relatives and patients, turning up late for theatre lists and rushing out the theatre door before the patient. He refused to participate in WHO Surgical Safety Checklists, and he was generally autocratic and rude. The CEO had already set a zero-tolerance agenda with his leadership team, and

---

99 Joint Commission (2008) *Behaviors that Undermine a Culture of Safety*. Sentinel Event Alert 40. Oakbrook Terrace, IL.

100 Rimmer A (2019) Poor teamwork among surgeons is affecting patient care, finds college. *BMJ* 364. Available at: www.bmj.com/content/364/bmj.l1371 (accessed August 2023).

he was bold. He went to the theatre, asked to speak to the surgeon (who was charming to the CEO, apparently), and told him to empty his locker as he was suspended forthwith and would not, he imagined, be returning, as he was being dismissed with immediate effect for gross misconduct.

That one action sent a very clear message to others who felt their position allowed them to behave as they wished, to prioritise their private practice and to treat staff badly. It also sent a message that the CEO and board would act if concerns were reported, and that they would protect staff from bullying. At that point the culture began to change, and in two years the service went from 'Inadequate' to a solid 'Good' rating. Staff absence reduced, care practice improved, patient feedback improved, and the number of incidents with harm reduced. Were the improvements linked to a leader that tackled inappropriate behaviour? I am absolutely sure they were.

Policy and governance

There should be evidence of checking compliance with the policies as part of the organisational governance. Some aspects of that are relatively straightforward – a regular check as to whether statutory notifications have been submitted to the CQC when a safeguarding referral has been made simply needs a tick in a box on a paper form or in an electronic check box. Other aspects are harder to build strong governance around; but this does not negate the need to do so, and the best providers will want to find ways to review the practice relating to consent and safeguarding. The way this will be done will depend on the provider, the size of the organisation and the scope of services provided. In most settings, there will be information recorded such as:

- Records of safeguarding supervision for key staff.
- Records of reflective discussion of safeguarding incidents both to support staff and to promote learning.
- An audit of safeguarding referrals to ensure that forms are completed and submitted promptly, and that there has been follow-up action if necessary.
- Training records for safeguarding and consent training at the correct levels for the role. There is published guidance available that offers comprehensive advice about the level of training required for staff working in healthcare settings.[101] There is also a wealth of information available to providers about safeguarding adults and the competency required. An online search engine will take you to pages of information, including the CQC website pages on safeguarding.[102] Training completion rates are rarely 100% because of staff movements, sickness or maternity leave, but they should be above a reasonable target. A very good provider

---

101 www.rcn.org.uk/Professional-Development/publications/pub-007366 (accessed June 2023)

102 www.cqc.org.uk/sites/default/files/20140416_safeguarding_adults_-_roles_and_responsibilities_-_revised_draf....pdf (accessed August 2023).

would meet a 95% target; most offer a 90% target, which some meet and some do not. The smaller the service, the greater the impact of a few staff not completing training. Two people from a staff of one hundred still gives a 98% completion rate compared to two people from a staff of ten where the rate falls to 80%. Mandatory training records should be current and show high levels of compliance with the required training.

■ In most services, there needs to be a training record that shows staff have been offered support around the Mental Capacity Act (2005) and its impact on the various roles which staff are employed in. It must include training in the Deprivation of Liberty Safeguards, so that staff are aware of most people's right to freedom to do as they wish – even old people!

■ Ideally, there should be compliance audits around the Mental Capacity Act (2005), to ensure that nobody is being subjected to restrictions unlawfully. That might be a paper exercise to check that, where restrictions have been imposed, the necessary process have been followed and there was Deprivation of Liberty Safeguards Approval. Better still might be someone walking around and looking to see whether there are any unnecessary restrictions on people's liberty. They'd need a checklist to follow or training in the specifics – were bedrails used, were doors to garden areas locked, had walking aids been moved away from the people that needed them and so on. If they found restrictions, they would need to follow up that they had been duly authorised and that the correct process had been followed. They would need to speak to people using the service about their life and the amount of choice they had, and to staff about how they minimised restrictions and supported choices. The visits would need to be recorded somehow (on the checklist, perhaps). Who should do the walk-arounds? It can be anyone who has been through appropriate recruitment processes to allow them unrestricted access to people using the service. Ideally, not the registered manager or a line manager, as they may hear what they want to hear, and people may not be entirely open with them. In an acute hospital, it could be a non-executive director, a suitable volunteer, a governor, a student nurse, a member of Healthwatch or someone from the Chaplaincy team. In a care home, it could be a peer-registered manager or team leader from another home in the group, a member of Healthwatch, a volunteer recruited to this task or a student social worker from the local university. It doesn't really matter who does it as long as they understand their remit and have access to the senior leaders to feed back their findings.

■ Closed culture reviews. Closed cultures can happen almost anywhere, but there are services and parts of services where the risks are higher and where there needs to be robust monitoring and steps to reduce the risks. In terms of documentary evidence, some is probably available, but not monitored for that specific purpose. If there is no use of that data by the provider, then it seems unreasonable to expect the CCQ staff on a short inspection to consider it. A wise provider of higher-risk services will ensure regular, open-minded documented reviews. Probably once a quarter or so, and preferably carried out by someone independent of the organisation. There may be visitor entry records that show that there are regular professional and family and friends visitors to the service, including at weekends and into the evening. There are staff rotas that can be scrutinised to make sure there are changes to who works with who, particularly on night shifts or other times when there are lower visitor numbers. There should be observation of care records by a senior member of staff as part of staff supervision. There should be records of regular contact between staff and family members or other representatives. There should be walk-around visits to the service or parts of the service by people slightly removed from care delivery, and these should include discussion with staff and people using the service. There should be Deprivation of Liberty Safeguard records and comprehensive records for anyone detained under the Mental Health Act with evidence of advocacy and independent review. Individual records should show oversight of wider needs, GP appointments, dental checks, activities, and visits from outside of the organisation. Complaints records will show if there have been complaints that indicate that a closed culture exists or is developing.

■ There needs to be documentary evidence that staff are supported to be kind and to exhibit positive behaviours, and that any allegations are investigated without prejudice and acted upon where findings show there has been unacceptable behaviour. Staff and people using the service need to feel safe talking about poor behaviours – they need to know that there will be no repercussions if the concerns were made in good faith, and that the behaviours will be addressed, even if the person they are raising concerns about is in a senior position. What can the documentary evidence be?

   ■ All organisations need to be clear what they stand for and what their overriding priorities and focus are. The staff need to know that from the point of recruitment. This means providers need a clear vision and a mission statement. It doesn't have to be complex or long, but it does need to give a message about what the service is and how it will be delivered. KFC offered a mission statement in 2013 that read, "To sell food in a fast, friendly environment that appeals to price-conscious, health-minded consumers...". The same year they had a mantra about appealing to health-minded consumers was the year they launched a burger that replaced the bun with fried chicken. Not ideal. Somewhat better is the statement from an American Psychiatric Hospital: "Because not all wounds are visible, we, are dedicated to healing the unseen. We do that by helping our patients overcome mental health challenges. We're committed to being confidential, sympathetic, and approachable in our communications and treatment." This statement sets a tone and cultural expectations in a few words. It sounds like somewhere I might want to be cared for or to work.

- An allegations policy that is known and followed is a good starting point in addressing allegations. A quick chat with a team leader who tells young female paramedics their bottom looks good in green and makes excuses to 'just squeeze past' is not sufficient to demonstrate to the young female paramedic that she is safe to raise concerns if the innuendo and creepy touching escalate into something more serious. She's likely to leave rather than see an assault dismissed by a regional manager who has known the team leader since he qualified and knows that he is a good chap, married with kids, an all-round top bloke.

- A behaviour framework that is explicit about expected behaviours and which is used during one-to-one supervision sessions, appraisals and incident review processes supports the policy. The documents that use the behaviour framework are evidence that behaviours are discussed, and that the staff are supported to reflect and consider behaviours.

- Referrals to professional bodies and records of disciplinary actions are another good form of evidence that poor behaviour is addressed.

- Staff surveys that ask specific questions about raising concerns about the behaviour of others and whether staff feel allegations would be dealt with. Obviously there needs to be visible action where there are issues raised.

- Time in team meetings, separate sessions or awaydays using reflective practice to discuss the impact of behaviours (perhaps through reviewing a complaint or an incident). Sometimes finding time for this sort of learning can be a challenge, but it is so important in building a positive culture.

- Walk-arounds that consider culture. Use someone who is comfortable asking about sensitive issues, and who is perceived as approachable and open to hearing hard messages. Speak to staff with protected characteristics about whether they have experienced homophobia, misogyny, racism, or other prejudiced behaviours. Look and listen in staff rooms for signs of prejudicial and intolerant behaviour – posters of topless women or 'banter' that tips over into bullying or racism. Record these so that you have evidence and, more importantly, so that staff know that such behaviours are not tolerated and will be addressed.

- Safeguarding referrals where people raised allegations of potential abuse or have signs or symptoms that have the potential to be deliberately inflicted. Individual records of proper decision-making if someone who is living with dementia makes frequent allegations about staff behaviours.

Evidence from staff and service users

The evidence from staff and people using the service will follow on from the documentary evidence. If the systems and processes to identify, monitor and react to safeguarding concerns and inappropriate behaviours are used effectively, then staff will tell the inspection team about them. If that young female paramedic was asked to speak to a female senior leader, supported by a Freedom to Speak up Guardian or friend, and she felt listened to and knew that the team leader had received a formal warning and agreed to mediation, then she is more likely to remain in service and more likely to tell others to report any concerns they share with her. She is also likely to tell the inspection team that she felt supported and that the issue was addressed. If staff have received good safeguarding training, then they will be able to tell the inspection team how they would react to someone sharing an allegation of abuse with them and talk about the reporting process within the service.

If the relatives of someone in a care home who is living with dementia have been asked about whether they feel able to raise concerns, they might say that they see the registered manager most times that they visit, and, if not the manager, then the deputy. They might say that the staff tell them about everything that happens, and so they know that a bruised and grazed shin was caused by their mother walking into a heavy wooden chair when coming indoors after doing some gardening.

If a parent lives a long way from their child who is a young adult living in a specialist learning disability service, they might say they never hear anything and it's difficult because they live so far away and their child is nonverbal – but last time they did go down the young person was on their own because they had developed very aggressive behaviour and needed two-to-one care on an isolation unit. They might point out they don't know why this has happened as the child was never aggressive at boarding school or at home. Alternatively, they might say that the staff are lovely and call every Friday evening with a weekly update. They might say the young adult had changed bedrooms as they didn't get along with a new resident who was in the bedroom next door and liked loud music. And they might say that the provider is very supportive and has a flat they can use to see their child more often and spend some weekends with them, doing things they enjoy and having the cuddles they miss so much.

It's a choice, isn't it – and one for the provider, not the parents or young person?

Chapter 14: Involving people to manage risks

Quality Statement:

We work with people to understand and manage risks by thinking holistically so that care meets their needs in a way that is safe and supportive and enables them to do the things that matter to them.

The idea behind this Quality Statement can be difficult to understand, because while we would all, I suspect, claim to be committed to personalised, holistic care, the reality of ensuring safe systems and delivering a service within financial and political constraints can drive us towards the opposite approach.

I always tell my now-adult children that we love them all the same but differently, and I have always adopted an approach of 'from each according to ability, to each according to needs.' That sounds Marxist, but it actually comes from the Bible. It's how we believe we should parent, even now. We did, of course, set boundaries that were common to all, and we looked carefully at the piles of Christmas presents before we wrapped them to ensure that there was fairness in cost. We didn't buy them all the same things, though – our son no more desired a violin upgrade or new pointed shoes than his sisters did some rugby under armour or an air rifle. Our son was supported (not entirely voluntarily, but in his best interests) to attend a tutorial programme in Oxford between Christmas and New Year to enable him to get decent grades in his A-levels, whereas his elder sister was very studious and needed support to ensure she had good work experience to support her expected high grades for university application.

Our youngest wanted to continue to dance throughout sixth form and, given the travel times to school and dance lessons, that was going to have an impact on outcomes, so we reluctantly supported her choice to board where she could continue to study hard and still pirouette and fondu as she wanted. That was a hard decision to make and was not without risks - homesickness, a totally new environment, handing over responsibility to the school, reduced oversight, and many other things that went through our minds before we agreed. The point is that everyone is different, and while there must be consistency and known expectations, there must also be consideration of personal preferences and the risks around individual choices.

People have a right to self-determination, and health and social care providers do not have the right to remove that without following due process. That process to restrict choice and the freedom to make decisions is enshrined in the Mental Capacity Act (2005) for anyone over sixteen years of age. Hopefully that doesn't come as a surprise to anyone reading this, but interpreting the Act can be a little harder. Most staff working in health and social care want to protect people from harm, and many think that their role is to keep people safe and make them better if they are ill. That is generally accepted as being what their roles are about, but there is a caveat that needs adding, which is: 'if they want to be kept safe or made better'. Most people do, of course, and most people are happy to take the advice and guidance of providers and their staff. After all, we consult with GPs because we want them to use their expertise to advise us about some aspect of ill health – usually.

Person-centred care, capacity and consent

This Quality Statement is about consent and person-centred care. It links to Regulation 12, which is about safe care and treatment. There is a valid argument that you cannot have safe care if the opportunity for truly informed consent has not been given – with all the risks and benefits compared, the procedures explained in detail, and the expected outcomes made clear.

Providing that level of detail when asking someone whether they want sugar in their tea is not really what this is about. Of course, there are risks associated with having four spoons of granulated added to each of the six cups of milky tea the service user enjoys every day, and there may well be scope for helping a young adult with a learning disability to understand that the reason they need to go to the dentist and have fillings is because of the sugar they consume. But, if they have the capacity to be supported to understand the risks of very high sugar intake, then the staff have no right to use sweeteners instead, thinking they are doing the right thing.

Not providing that level of detail when someone is deciding whether to agree to treatment having been diagnosed with an early prostate cancer, however, is clearly wrong. Men in this situation must fully understand the options, risks and benefits. It may be that they are comfortable with a 'wait and watch' approach, having regular PSA blood tests to indicate if there is an increasing risk. Others, though, might feel that they would struggle to live knowing that a cancer was lurking inside them and would want surgery. The risks of surgery are not insignificant, and the person needs to be made aware of the level of risk around impotence and incontinence, both of which could be life-changing for a man in his fifties with a successful career. He needs to have every treatment option explained with hard data around the level of risk – and the decision, while guided by the urologist, should be his alone to make. The urologist's role is simply to supply accurate information and address any concerns.

It is harder when someone is unable, even with support, to make important decisions for themselves. How then do providers ensure that they are considering the person's preferences and wishes? In some areas of care provision it is relatively easy, although challenges can happen in unexpected ways and need careful consideration at the time.

The first principle that needs to be adhered to is the assumption that people have capacity to make their own decisions. No service should be deferring to relatives, even those with a Lasting Power of Attorney, where a person has capacity or could be supported to make their own decision. If a person living in a care home says they want a glass of wine with their lunch, usually they should be allowed to do so. The person's daughter or son might tell the staff that they aren't to be allowed it because they are a Muslim family and alcohol is Haram – against the laws of Islam. It might be easier to accept this opinion, but is it right? What if the staff didn't offer wine but the person still asked for it? What if they took someone else's wine if they weren't offered any? Whose decision is paramount? Is the risk in allowing someone with reduced capacity to change what was an accepted choice for them previously, or in allowing them to make a decision when they have reduced capacity?

In every service type there are wonderful examples of staff 'going the extra mile' to personalise care and ensure that people's needs are met. However, there are also restrictions imposed where none are really necessary and where those restrictions impact on the way people experience care and treatment. A particular 'bee in my bonnet' is people being accompanied to the operating theatre. It is now the norm that parents can accompany children to theatre and wait while they are anaesthetised. It is better for the child, because operating theatres can be scary places if you are seven years old, and a parental presence can offer reassurance and a sense of safety. Children are more likely to be compliant and settled if a parent is with them, and that is better for staff, too. Screaming children create stress, stress leads to tension that can increase mistakes, and that is not good in an operating theatre. Yet not all countries accept parents in the anaesthetic area, and there is research from Canada as late as 2018 showing that, while parents want to be there, sometimes medical professionals are less keen.[103] That is about meeting the needs of the staff, and perpetuating a system where the child's and parent's preferences are secondary. In a similar way, in maternity units across the country, fathers are often present during caesarean sections and provide reassurance and a sense of safety for the mother, as well as being able to see or hold their baby at a very early stage.

Frightened adults (and children over sixteen) usually have to cope alone, in a room of strangers wearing masks and with strange noises around them. What is the difference between a frightened seventeen-year-old and a frightened fifteen-year-old? And it isn't only in theatres (where I accept it

---

103 Yousef Y, Drudi S, Maria Sant'Anna A & Emil S (2018) Parental presence at induction of anesthesia: perceptions of a pediatric surgical department before and after program implementation. *Journal of Pediatric Surgery* 53 (8). Available at: www.sciencedirect.com/science/article/abs/pii/S0022346818300162 (accessed August 2023).

might be inconvenient but not insurmountable to have someone alongside the patient) – it is also quite often during the time beforehand, in day surgery units. People are asked to arrive around 7am, before the start of the list, and may not be taken to theatre for several hours. Often, they are not allowed someone with them because it is inconvenient for the staff, so they are left sitting around with very little to do, anxious and thirsty. Often, they are asked to put a gown on and sit around in a dressing gown as well. The pathway could be changed if we decided to keep people using services as the focus. Pagers are available nowadays, so that some people could go for a walk and be paged half hour before their theatre slot, thus increasing space in the pre-operative area, reducing stress for people and allowing them to have someone with them. Staff would then have more time to focus on those patients that really needed their support.

Inclusion and inequality

This Quality Statement also links to Regulation 10, which is about dignity and respect. The guidance says that all communication with people using services must be respectful, and that this includes using or facilitating the most suitable means of communication – as well as respecting a person's right to choose whether or not to engage in communication. Language can often be a barrier and many, many reports from the Commission, particularly those relating to acute healthcare settings, simply say that the staff had access to a telephone interpreting system. However, healthcare professionals will often say that the telephone interpreting is never available, and that they don't use it because it is too complicated to set up a call with a live translator. Often staff say they use a search engine translation service on their personal phones and that helps, or they say that they use relatives or friends.

Recent reports suggest that inspection teams show limited consideration of compliance with this regulation, and that the narrative is, at best, limited. A recent inspection report of an ear-syringing service simply said that: "Staff communicated with people in a way that they could understand, for example, communication aids and easy read materials were available". There was nothing about how people with hearing loss were supported, and nothing about people with a limited understanding of English. A care home report published around the same time said that "Staff were knowledgeable about people's communication needs, for example, a staff member told us they had to repeat things several times for a person to help them understand." I think this state of events is likely to change, and in future there will be a greater focus on how people are communicated with – simply because it has such a significant impact on their ability to give informed consent, on the respect staff are showing them and on the safety of the service.

Clearly, the Commission has some work to do to ensure that it regulates in a way which ensures that all people are offered the safety of informed consent and the risk reduction that dignified and person-centred care offers. There is much work going on around this, and it is one of the benefits that the single assessment framework will hopefully bring. Just as care homes must ensure that they find ways for people who have limited understanding of English to engage fully and to give their consent (where they have capacity), so too other services will have to produce evidence of how they do this – and simply having a contract with an online interpreting service may not be sufficient.

The Commission has a core ambition running through its Strategic Objectives that is about tackling inequalities in health and care – pushing for equality of access, experiences and outcomes from health and social care services.[104] It would be very difficult to realise that ambition without placing a greater focus on equality of access, experiences and outcomes in the inspection process. The Commission lays claim to a commitment to its ambition of regulating to advance equality and protect people's Human Rights. It says that everyone in health and social care has a role to play in tackling the inequalities in health and care for some people, and how providers are playing their part is likely to be determined through the inspection process. Increasingly, then, providers will be asked to demonstrate how they are meeting people's needs relating to protected characteristics, and how they are identifying and responding to health and care inequalities.

We know that black women are five times more likely to die during childbirth as white women in the UK.[105] That is a very concerning statistic. But too often it can be dismissed as just that, a statistic. A worrying one that is talked about in meetings and put on databases, but which fails to show the tragedy and pain caused by these lost lives. The reasons are multifactorial, and we know some of the factors that lead to worse outcomes for black mothers and babies, but the changes to address these factors and make outcomes more equal aren't often made. I am sure that is the same with other areas of care, and for others with a protected characteristic.

One factor is that black women's pain is not always reacted to in the same way as white women's pain, and is underestimated. One mother who gave birth in 2015 says that her pain was underestimated – and she believes the colour of her skin played into this. She said, "Within way less time than I was advised my contractions kicked in hard and fast. When I called a nurse for pain relief, they advised me to 'take a warm bath with lavender'." The young mother recalls barely being able to walk to the bathroom from

104 CQC (2022) *A new strategy for the changing world of health and social care* [online]. Available at www.cqc.org.uk/about-us/our-strategy-plans/new-strategy-changing-world-health-social-care-cqcs-strategy-2021 (accessed August 2023).

105 Knight M, Bunch K, Tuffnell D, Jayakody H, Shakespeare J, Kotnis R, Kenyon S & Kurinczuk JJ (Eds.) (2018) on behalf of MBRRACE-UK. Saving Lives, Improving Mothers' Care – Lessons learned to inform maternity care from the UK and Ireland Confidential Enquiries into Maternal Deaths and Morbidity 2014-16. Oxford: National Perinatal Epidemiology Unit, University of Oxford.

her bed because the pain was so bad. She remembers getting into the bath unassisted, and fighting the urge to pass out from the pain due to another contraction coming in fast and strong. Despite being in complete agony and alone, and demanding pain relief of any sort (she had opted for an epidural in her birth plan), she was told to breathe through the contractions.

Another factor is that black women are more likely to have additional complicating health factors, some of which are related to living in poverty – and evidence shows that poverty persistence is much more prevalent for Black and Minority Ethnic groups, who are between two and three times more likely to be in persistent poverty than people in white families. For example, three in ten people (28%) living in families with a mixed/multiple ethnic head of household are in persistent poverty, compared to 10% of those living in families with a white head of household.[106] Health and social care providers may not have the ability to address the poverty they see, but they can adjust their services to accommodate and consider the needs of people who live in poverty. In maternity care, a middle-class mother travelling to a consultant appointment will probably drive or have her partner drive her while her children are at nursery or cared for by granny. A poor mother may have to find someone to care for her other children, use public transport and find the money for the ticket. She is likely to arrive stressed, and may not take in everything she is told as she is worrying about getting home before her neighbour has to collect her own children from school. There are all sorts of ways in which the poorer mother, with greater difficulties accessing services, can be supported to get the right care.

Guidance provided by the UK Government in the 2022 report *Health Disparities and Health Inequalities: Applying All Our Health* says "In England, there is a nineteen-year gap in healthy life expectancy (whether we experience health conditions or diseases that impact how long we live in good health) between the most and least affluent areas of the country, with people in the most deprived neighbourhoods, certain ethnic minority and inclusion health groups getting multiple long-term health conditions ten to fifteen years earlier than the least deprived communities, spending more years in ill health and dying sooner."[107] That is quite an indictment of our society. Many types of health and social care providers and leaders need to be able to demonstrate that they have considered what they can do to address this problem, and to improve outcomes for all. Many do not even collate data by ethnicity or protected characteristics – I have yet to see an incident report or board paper that shows the ethnicity of a baby or mother,

---

106 SMC (2020) *Measuring Poverty 2020* [online]. Available at: https://socialmetricscommission. org.uk/wp-content/uploads/2020/06/Measuring-Poverty-2020-Web.pdf (accessed August 2023).

107 Gov.uk (2022) *Health Disparities and Health Inequalities: Applying All Our Health* [online]. Available at: www.gov.uk/government/publications/health-disparities-and-health-inequalities-applying-all-our-health/health-disparities-and-health-inequalities-applying-all-our-health (accessed August 2023).

and I am not yet convinced that it is seen as part of the review process. The Commission's focus on health inequalities and different outcomes for different groups will likely see pressure applied to collect and consider data such as the rate of incidents by ethnicity. It should not take a regulator to make this happen; good providers will want to do it.

Needs and preferences

Inequalities are not just about acute healthcare. All providers need to reflect on their service delivery and ensure that people are receiving care and treatment that reflects their needs and preferences. Commissioners should be ensuring that services are commissioned in a way that allows greater equity of access and outcomes. That might mean ensuring the tissue-viability policy and training supports staff to recognise changes to darker skin that might be indicative of pressure damage. The usual redness may be less apparent, and staff need to be aware of this when caring for people who may be at risk of pressure damage.

Similarly, people who are deaf may need some adaptation along with the provision of sign language interpreters, changed seating positions to enable lip reading, or other measures that help them understand and react to information. Writing it down may be necessary in an emergency department, but having staff who can sign a little is preferable. It can be done. When I last visited the critical care unit at St Richard's Hospital in West Sussex, the staff were caring for a young deaf man after a serious road traffic accident. His wife was also deaf. Several of the staff had learned to sign. Not whole conversations, but enough to allow the patient and his wife to feel included and to show that they cared enough to bother. At the other end of the spectrum, I recall a provider of a diagnostic imaging service who claimed they had disabled access because there was a ramp into the shared entrance to the premises from the street and so people using a wheelchair could be accommodated. When I asked how someone with very restricted mobility would get from their wheelchair to the couch, they didn't know.

There are far too many individual needs to cover in one book or on one inspection. Providers and registered managers need to understand their service, and who might need or want to use it, and make provision to enable that. They also need to consider people's needs and preferences when planning care. That planning needs to be in discussion with the person using the service, and with the assumption that they have capacity unless there is evidence to the contrary.

If someone appears to lack capacity to make a specific decision, then providers need to ensure that they operate within the requirements of the Mental Capacity Act (2005) and either work with someone who has a registered Lasting Power of Attorney or make a legitimate best interest decision. If someone needs an interpreter, easy read documents, signing, or other adaptations and support to help them make the decision, then that should be provided. If a person has capacity, then any decision involving their health and social care is theirs to make – even if it is unwise, odd, not what staff think should happen, unpopular or high risk. The caveats are around legality and safeguarding where there may be a requirement for staff to intervene. In most cases, even legality is down to the person with capacity – if someone wants to travel on a train without a ticket, they have the right to do so knowing that they are likely to face sanctions through the courts. If they want to drive a car having consumed a bottle of wine, however, then the need to keep others safe overrides the right to drive and it would be perfectly appropriate to involve the police.

Most adults can decide their own risk threshold. We all do it when pulling out at junctions, skydiving, swimming in the sea in November or climbing Mont Blanc. In 2012, Sister Madonna Buder, a nun, competed in her final 'Ironman' competition in Canada, aged eight-two. She was still competing in marathons aged ninety. At ninety-two, Paul Spangler finished his fourteenth marathon. Good social care providers support people using their services to take risks in measured ways, as long as they understand the possible consequences. Healthcare providers more often have to ensure that people are aware of the risks of refusing or delaying treatment.

All those scenarios should be covered in the Consent or Mental Capacity Policy. They are key documents that must be available and understood by all staff. Having the policy is not enough – staff must enact it every time they interact with people using the service. Nurses should not simply tell people that they must put on a hospital gown; they should explain the reasons why it may be advisable. If a woman having a hysteroscopy knows that lots of water is involved, they may be more willing to take their dress off and use the gown provided. That is a reasonable ask. Staff in the emergency department telling someone they must put on a gown as there are no changing facilities in the x-ray area and it slows staff down so they get cross is a less reasonable request, and a refusal should be accepted. Staff need to understand that people can refuse whatever they want, assuming they have capacity. Consent forms and consent form audits are good evidence that there is proper consideration of people's right to make their own decisions.

Do Not Attempt Cardio-Pulmonary Resuscitation (DNACPR)

There also needs to be a resuscitation policy or other titled policy that covers the organisational stance on decisions around whether to attempt resuscitation and the way staff should determine the level of care to be provided. It is not appropriate for any single healthcare professional to determine how those decisions will be made, as there is too much scope for conscious and unconscious bias around the emergency care of someone with a protected characteristic and assumptions about quality of life based on an individual's own narrow perspective. There must be clear guidance, known to staff, about who can make decisions and how this is to be done.

Properly completed Do Not Attempt Cardio-Pulmonary Resuscitation (DNACPR) forms are a good source of evidence and will usually be looked at (while they might well be part of a wider assessment of advanced planning or ReSPECT forms, the DNACPR is still something that will be considered).[108] The Commission reviewed the use of DNACPR forms and decision-making during the pandemic, and published a report of the findings entitled 'Protect, respect, connect – decisions about living and dying well during COVID-19'.[109] I would recommend that providers and staff look at it, as it makes for sad reading. The report says that some people felt that conversations around whether they would want to receive CPR came out of the blue, and that they were not given the time or information to fully understand what was happening or even what a DNACPR was. In some cases, people were not even aware that a DNACPR decision was in place.

The decision-making around DNACPR is complex, and many health and social care staff have a limited grasp of it, so it is no wonder that many people using services and their families also find it hard to understand. People talk about consenting to a DNACPR when the reality is that one cannot consent to not having resuscitation. One can only consent to something that does happen. What providers and leaders need to be able to demonstrate is that the person is included in the discussions, that the reasons why resuscitation might not be appropriate are made clear, and that there is wider discussion around the desired and appropriate ceiling of care and action in the event of a sudden deterioration in someone's condition. What the evidence obtained from looking at completed, individual DNACPR forms should not show is cohorting of the decisions and a lack of consideration of the individual. The reasons section of a DNACPR form should *not* simply have 'learning disability' or 'progressive disease' as the sole determiner of whether someone is actively treated in the event of their heart stopping. Age shouldn't be a particular determiner of whether to attempt resuscitation, but a person's level of frailty must. Frailer people are more like to die during, or soon after, treatment, and may lose the opportunity to say goodbye to loved ones or make peace with their God.

There needs to be consideration of what the person wants – and they should be encouraged to involve their families or partners in this discussion, so they are supported to be heard. Too often, people are not given a voice because their default setting is to do what the doctor suggests. Those discussions need

---

108 www.resus.org.uk/respect (accessed August 2023).
109 www.cqc.org.uk/sites/default/files/20210318_dnacpr_printer-version.pdf (accessed August 2023).

to be recorded. Not necessarily verbatim, but in sufficient detail to ensure that there is evidence of who has been involved and what the discussion outcomes were. That is partly about inspection and accountability, but it is also protective of the healthcare professionals involved, in the event of distressed family members raising concerns through their grief.

The Commission offers guidance around advanced decision-making and planning for emergency care and treatment. In its 'GP Mythbusters', the CQC recognises that staff need training and says, "DNACPR decisions and conversations should be undertaken by members of the healthcare team who are appropriately trained, competent and experienced. Training should give health and care professionals the knowledge, skills and confidence to talk to the patient and their relatives or carers about advance care planning and DNACPR decisions."

Providers therefore need to be able to demonstrate that there has been training for the people who are involved in DNACPR decisions. That means GPs and doctors of all grades working in areas of the NHS where there is a likelihood of those discussions by doctors of their grade. A relatively junior doctor in an emergency department or elderly care ward may require that training, but it should fall to a consultant to have the conversation about a child with a terminal illness. There should be training not only in the process and legalities, but also in how to approach the conversation. A barked "There is little point in attempting resuscitation" directed towards relatives sitting beside their aged parent who has had a major stroke in an emergency department is callous, and it can never be normalised regardless of how busy the department is. Doctors need training to make a difficult conversation better for everyone.

Other types of providers must have training that meets the needs of the people using their service. An independent hospital may or may not need to train their doctors to have DNACPR discussions if they offer, perhaps, cancer care or long-term care of people with advanced neurological conditions. Somewhere only offering elective orthopaedic surgery would usually not need their resident medical officers to be having those conversations, as that discussion should fall to the person's GP who is more aware of their holistic needs and condition.

Care home staff, paramedics, community nurses, learning disabilities nurses and mental health nurses all need training around the provider's DNACPR policy. They may not (and should not, usually) be the decision-makers, but they need to know what the form means for them and the people they are caring for. They need to know when to challenge, when to ask for the form to be completed properly and, importantly, what the limitations of care are. They really need to understand that a DNACPR is only about resuscitation in the event of someone's heart stopping, rather than stopping the treatment of reversible conditions.

Hospice doctors would usually be very comfortable discussing the subject of DNACPR and have real expertise in this area. Rarely would inpatient hospice doctors need to have the conversation, unless another doctor had been derelict in their responsibilities. Sometimes, hospice doctors need to reinforce the information and offer repeated explanations to patients or relatives. They need to help people understand why prescribing antibiotics by intravenous injection is okay, but using a defibrillator is not. Usually, they are pretty good at that, and they can be a useful source of support and advice to other providers within their local system.

There must be records of DNACPR training, and the DNACPR policy needs to say how often the training must be repeated. The training will vary for different professions and grades of staff, and the records should demonstrate that too.

Other policies

In terms of other policies, they need to be sufficient to mitigate the specific risks related to each service type, and training records must show that there has been training around those risks. There are too many possibilities to be detailed in a book, but it might be that a private surgery provider specifically excludes anyone who lacks the capacity to make their own decision around elective surgery that is available on the NHS, as paying for treatment that is available for free may not be in their best interest. Or it might be that there is a need for a policy around the use of electric mobility scooters by residents in a care home, or perhaps a policy around visiting hours and priorities for use of single rooms in an NHS service.

Regardless of what the policy relates to, every policy should contain details of how the service is considering how the policy affects different individuals and groups, particularly those with protected characteristics. That might mean making sure that the consent policy requires a British Sign Language Interpreter when someone who is deaf is being offered cosmetic surgery, or that there is an easy read document and possibly a Makaton interpreter when discussing end-of-life care arrangements with someone with a learning disability.

Thinking about a few specific practices and personal preferences, it is worth providers considering requests for same-sex health care professionals and carers. The law is not specific in this regard, and there are conflicting needs of different patient groups and staff groups, but the Local Government Ombudsman passed a judgement in 2014 that, under the Equality Act (2010), the need to deliver same-sex care is an 'objective justification' for advertising and recruiting workers to fulfil the need.[110] It is not enough for a provider to

---

110 www.lgo.org.uk/information-centre/news/2014/nov/not-providing-same-sex-carers-can-impact-dignity-says-ombudsman (accessed August 2023).

say, "We cannot guarantee same-sex care." They need to demonstrate that they have made every effort to ensure the service is delivered in the way that is best for the recipient.

In every service I have worked in or with, the needs of people wanting same-sex care has rarely been prioritised or practiced. Sometimes it can be difficult; in an emergency department the only consultant available may be a different sex to the patient, and that may mean they have to decide whether to accept care from someone of the opposite sex or decline care. Assuming capacity, it is their right to make that decision, and because it is sometimes unavoidable in hospitals and GP practices, providers should have a chaperone policy. That needs to consider individual needs, and people acting as chaperones need training, as with other policies. I have yet to see care homes provide chaperones for people having intimate care by a same-sex carer. Is this because older people, particularly those living with dementia, are often not considered to deserve the same level of respect and dignity, I wonder?

Given that the adult social care workforce is made up of around 82% female workers, there should be no need for women to have a male carer provide intimate care – and certainly not without another member of the care staff team or a chaperone present. It may be harder for smaller care providers to offer same-sex care to men residing at a home, but it should certainly be a consideration. There are real risks (that we don't like talking about) of male carers working alone with female service users in community settings. That is not to say all males working in the care industry or in healthcare are abusive, far from it, but given that there were 35,606 'sexual safety incidents' recorded in hospitals between 2017 and 2022 by NHS Trusts in England, it is something that providers should probably be considering and a risk that needs mitigation.[111] Three-quarters of the reports were made in Mental Health Trusts, and nearly 2,500 of the alleged incidents of sexual violence and misconduct were by staff on patients.

There is a similar known concern in social care settings, with a report published in 2020 showing that the CQC received 661 statutory notifications from care providers describing 899 sexual incidents between March and May of 2018. Nearly 60% of the incidents were alleged to be carried out by people using the services, while 16% were alleged to be carried out by employed staff or visiting workers and in 8% of cases it was friends or relatives. That's forty-eight incidents of sexual abuse by staff reported each month, and of course it doesn't include those not identified or reported.

Only around 11% of nurses are male; it remains one of the most gender segregated of all professions. Why, then (my personal question), are men

111 Bawden A & Batty D (2023) *NHS England mental health trusts record 26,000 sexual abuse incidents* [online]. Available at: www.theguardian.com/society/2023/may/23/nhs-england-mental-health-trusts-record-26000-sexual-abuse-incidents (accessed August 2023).

working on gynaecology wards and in female bays or wards? It won't be a universally popular view, and I present it as a point for providers to reflect on rather than, necessarily, an assertion of best practice. It is not my role to tell providers how to provide their service, after all. In shortage areas, it may be necessary to have care and treatment from someone of the opposite sex, but there is no shortage of female nurses, is there? Mammography screening is carried out in an all-female environment, so the idea is not new. Some men who are nurses report enjoying their time on gynaecology wards, but the service is not being provided for them – or at least it shouldn't be.

The focus should be on women having protection from male perpetrators, because men are responsible for around 98% of all sexual offences in the UK – and we know that offences happen in social care and hospital settings. While most men of course do not offend, the likelihood is far greater where there is a man providing care. Abusers focus on the vulnerable, and those in social care settings are very vulnerable indeed.

Same-sex accommodation has been a longstanding requirement in the NHS, with the 2019 guidance saying that:

"…providers of NHS-funded care are expected to have a zero-tolerance approach to mixed-sex accommodation, except where it is in the overall best interest of all patients affected. Patients should not normally have to share sleeping accommodation with members of the opposite sex. Patients should not have to share toilet or bathroom facilities with members of the opposite sex. Patients should not have to walk through an area occupied by patients of the opposite sex to reach toilets or bathrooms; this excludes corridors. Women-only day rooms should be provided in mental health inpatient units."[112]

That all seems perfectly reasonable and is usually not an issue, although breaches continue to be reported as demand increases and hospital capacity reduces. However, when a service really begins to think about the needs and preferences of different groups in fine detail, things can become somewhat more difficult.

For example, a non-binary person who was born a male may choose to be accommodated on a female ward in line with the NHS guidance. While this may meet their preferences, it may also be very distressing to women on the ward to be sharing sleeping and lavatory facilities with someone with the physical appearance of a man. Transgender women and non-binary people are protected under the Equality Act (2010) – but so are women, as sex is also a protected characteristic. A young nun, an orthodox Jewish woman or

---

112 NHS (2019) Delivering same-sex accommodation [online]. Available at: www.england.nhs. uk/statistics/wp-content/uploads/sites/2/2021/05/NEW-Delivering_same_sex_accommodation_ sep2019.pdf (accessed August 2023).

a Muslim woman may all find it distressing to see male genitalia and to be in their nightwear around people with male genitalia they are not related to. Empathising with a woman who has been subject to prior sexual abuse or assault, and who requests women-only health care staff, may also present a need to determine how best each person's needs are met.

Many maternity units offer fathers the opportunity to stay overnight on postnatal wards, which for some women is a really positive thing and for others is a concern. Midwives also have mixed views, unsurprisingly. In 2020, a group of midwives at Edinburgh's Royal Infirmary complained to NHS Lothian about fathers of new babies staying overnight in the hospital. They said it was putting strain on staff who claimed fathers "treat the ward like a hotel." They said that partners were sharing beds, ordering takeaways and using staff kitchens. One of their concerns was that some new mothers were too embarrassed to breastfeed or get changed because there were so many men staying at the postnatal unit.

On any ward, some mothers will want their partners there, some will be indifferent, and some will feel uncomfortable sleeping and changing with men nearby when their bodies are leaking and they are still adjusting to post-birth changes. The very best providers will recognise that there are differing preferences and needs, and will adjust the service they provide to accommodate these variances.

Evidence to support the Quality Statement

How can you evidence that the risks around personal dignity, feeling safe and having their privacy respected are being addressed and that the needs of people using the service are put above the needs or preferences of the staff?

Evidence from data and records

Clearly, individual care records are a good starting point. They all contain assessments around pressure damage risk, malnutrition risk, falls and mobility risk. Care assessments and care plans should also document the person's preferences around choice and, in some services, the risk threshold they are happy to live by. A care home provider might need to consider whether a person has the capacity to leave the home alone to go into the village, but they have no right to make any decision or attempt to impose limitations around what a person does there when there is no concern around capacity. In other words, care home staff cannot usually decide that a person can go and have a coffee and use the library in the local town, but they cannot go into a pub and buy a pint of beer (or even two, if they so choose).

Where there is reduced capacity, there is a need for individual records to show that there have been best interest decisions. For example, a twenty-two-year-old with Prader-Willi syndrome moving into residential care may lack the capacity to restrict their own food intake, or to understand the consequences of this. This means that there needs to be evidence of a mental capacity assessment by a suitably qualified person, not an old-school report or the parents saying they don't really understand food. It also means that there probably needs to be a best interest decision and a Deprivation of Liberty Safeguards approval from the local authority, to ensure that any decisions are being made in the young adult's best interests and are the least restrictive measures possible.

The best interest decision cannot simply be the parents telling the care staff that they have locks on the kitchen door at home and serve all their food on a plate at set times. Nor can it be the care home staff deciding that this is the easiest course of action and what they do for all the young people they work with, for various reasons. It must be a formally recorded best interest decision involving the young person, their family, the care home staff, and others with responsibilities for the health and wellbeing of the young person. That might mean consulting with the GP, the endocrinologist at the local hospital, the social worker and learning disabilities team and an independent mental capacity advocate. The young person's individual record needs to have the agreed minutes of that meeting, or other documentary evidence of the discussion and the involved parties who agreed the decision. Acting without the documentary evidence and restricting someone's freedoms without proper authority to do so is a serious breach of regulation.

If a service is accepting the decisions of someone claiming Lasting Power of Attorney (LPA), then there needs to be evidence in the individual's records that the donation of the Lasting Power of Attorney for health and welfare has been registered. Asking the person who claims to have LPA is insufficient – there needs to be a copy of the letter showing that the LPA is registered.

Providers can supplement the review of individual records by providing evidence of their own reviews and audits. In a very small service, nearly all the records may be looked at whereas in a large service only a small proportion can ever be scrutinised. If an inspection team looks at six records and there are minor shortcomings identified in four of them, then the report may read that the majority of records reviewed were incomplete. Unless evidence is found that this is not the case, and that the provider has regularly monitored the quality of recording with audits showing that compliance with the provider's recording policy is in fact much better than was seen in the sample, the findings cannot be challenged. If, however, there are monthly audits that show that records around mental capacity assessment and best interest decisions are compliant with the provider's policy 87% of the time, then the word 'majority' switches from the proportion that were not compliant to the proportion that were compliant. This approach to monitoring applies to all records, regardless of subject. If there is a policy about something then it usually needs monitoring and reviewing, either through a documentation audit or through observational audits.

Sometimes, carrying out audits and reviews can result in service changes that make life easier for staff. Not too long ago, anyone who was admitted to hospital had a fluid balance chart at the end of their bed. I suspect this is still the case in some settings with an overinsistence on underused charts that serve no particular purpose! There are times when monitoring fluid balance closely is essential, lifesaving even, and certainly a good indicator of the physiological state of someone who has been very unwell or as a tool to prevent harm being caused by excess fluids. Quite often, though, they are not necessary; few social care settings really need them unless there are concerns about an individual's risk of dehydration. Many hospital patients don't need them either; there should be clinical guidelines or a policy document around fluid balance for adult inpatients, with separate guidance for staff working with babies and children, giving the criteria for when fluid-balance charts should be used.

An audit of fluid-balance charts might well show that the compliance rates are low because there is limited compliance with the initiation criteria, and they were being used as a default setting. Perhaps staff see that they aren't needed, so they are only occasionally and vaguely completed. Simply writing 'cup of tea' or 'wet pad' gives very little useful information. An inspection team won't be looking to see whether the patients have fluid charts in accordance with the clinical guideline criteria; many don't have a clinical background. They will see that seven forms were not completed or totalled and extrapolate this to suggest that people were at risk of dehydration. Maybe access to end-of-bed electronic records will reduce the burden of unnecessary forms that aren't completed properly, and so provide evidence of care and practice shortfalls for something that wasn't needed in the first place.

Evidence from staff and service users

What will people using the service be asked? What evidence can services provide to show that people using the service are listened to and their wishes respected?

The sorts of questions that people using the service may be asked will differ depending on the service type. It would be odd to ask someone with a learning disability about how pain was managed, or whether they had spent time in a corridor after admission. However, I would hope they were asked about how they are supported to contribute to their community, to take part in activities that bring them pleasure and to make choices about how they live their life. Care home residents may be asked whether people knock on doors and wait for an answer before entering; or about whether they can have a lie-in or stay up to watch a late programme. They might be asked whether anyone has discussed with them their future care and what might happen if they became very unwell, and about the explanations they have had to help them with such decisions. Consent will certainly be talked about and observed – about little things, such as where someone wants to sit at lunchtime or what they want to wear, as well as sometimes (and in some services) around bigger decisions such as relationships and treatment choices.

Staff will be asked about their understanding of consent and the Mental Capacity Act (2005), with an expectation that they will have sufficient knowledge to carry out their role safely and in a way that is compliant with the law. They will be asked about how decisions are made and what restrictions are placed on people using the service. There may be questions about how people are involved in the delivery of the service, whether they have a say in activities and house rules. People using the service will likely be asked to answer the same sorts of questions from their perspective.

As with all areas of practice, the people being asked – whether they are staff, service users, their families or visiting professionals – will usually be honest. And if the service is a good one, where people are treated with respect and dignity, and they are allowed to make choices as appropriate, then more often than not they will say so.

Chapter 15: Safe environments

Quality Statement:

We detect and control potential risks in the care environment. We make sure that the equipment, facilities and technology support the delivery of safe care.

On the surface this seems like quite an easy Quality Statement to evidence – and it should be, as mostly is about having records of checks of premises and equipment. Failing to consistently meet statutory requirements, however, can result in lowered ratings or enforcement. As with most of the Quality Statements, it is really about what people do and fail to do – those acts of commission or omission by staff who, for whatever reason, don't do the checks that are meant to be done.

There are prosecutions for equipment failures in registered services, of course, but they are often prosecutions brought by other agencies. That doesn't diminish the need for providers to maintain oversight of premises and equipment safety, or to reduce the possibility of enforcement by the Commission. In any case, the question of who takes enforcement action isn't really important – the potential harm caused to people using services is what really matters.

In 2017, an eighty-five-year-old resident of a Manchester care home, who was living with dementia, was using the home's lift with a care worker. While they were in it, the lift stopped for a few seconds before plunging four metres into the basement. The resident died following the fall, and the care worker sustained minor injuries. The investigation by the Health and Safety Executive found that the accident was due to poor maintenance; the corner of one of the lift's doors had been damaged, and it caught on the lintel plate of the ground floor landing entrance, causing it to bend and then buckle under its own weight, before dropping uncontrolled to the basement. The damaged door had been reported to the care home's lift-maintenance provider a week prior to the accident. However, while engineers had attended on the same day, they found that a replacement part was required, and therefore no repair had taken place at the time of the incident. Engineers also visited the home on the day of the incident for a scheduled maintenance visit, but they did not repair the door and the lift remained in use.

The court heard that, despite being fully aware of ongoing issues with the lift, the provider had not ensured that there was a system in place to deal with reports of defects, and it had not taken the necessary steps to rectify the issues identified. In 2021, the lift maintenance company was fined £14,400 and ordered to pay £45,000 costs following the accident. However, the court ruled that the care home itself was also responsible for the safe operation of the lift. The company which ran the home went into liquidation shortly after criminal proceedings started. This was the second such incident within a three-month period. The owner of a different care home was fined £90,000 after a care home manager fell down a lift shaft at the home.

There are clearly repercussions if providers do not ensure safe maintenance of their premises and equipment, or if they are not able to demonstrate that safety processes have been followed. In the scenario above, the provider had carried out six-monthly lift examination reports, as required by law, but these had not been provided to the lift maintenance company. How difficult is it to add a box on a lift inspection report that says, 'send to maintenance company'?

There are far too many examples of providers who have caused harm and even avoidable deaths because of failures to properly maintain equipment. In 2021, two nursing-home owners were ordered to pay £140,000 after a pensioner died following a fall from a hoist. The person fell while being moved from her bed to a chair at the home. She banged her head and died the next day. The Crown Court was told that the defective fifteen-year-old hoist was in such poor condition that it could not be used safely, and that it had not been properly inspected regularly. The hoist sling had a two-year lifespan, but it had been in use for nine. A replacement hoist sling is much cheaper and easier to deal with than a premature death and a £140,000 fine.

Managing self-harm risks

Ligature points are cited in many deaths and attempts by people to take their own lives. A ligature point is anything capable of bearing the whole or partial weight of a person which could be used to attach a cord, rope, or other material to for the purpose of hanging or strangulation. In a ward environment, ligature points can include shower rails, coat hooks, pipes and radiators, bedsteads, window and door frames, ceiling fittings, handles, hinges and closures. They do not have to be attached to a ceiling or high up; often such ligature points are low-lying. CCQ staff working with mental health services will always check whether environmental risk assessments have been completed, and whether potential ligature points have been removed from areas accessible by people at risk of attempting to harm themselves. This message is being spread across other services, as more people in mental health crisis are being cared for in acute hospital settings, particularly in emergency care departments and increasingly in services for children and young people. In truth, all providers need to consider the risk and ensure they minimise the possibility of anyone attempting or completing suicide when using their service.

In 2021, a Mental Health Trust was fined £1.5 million because it failed to "prevent suicide". The Trust pleaded guilty to an offence under the Health and Safety at Work Act (1974), following an investigation that identified eleven deaths where a point of ligature was used within a ward environment. The financial punishment is less hard-hitting than the words of the mother of a young man who died aged twenty. She described the moment she was told the news, saying "a part of me died with him". "Every day is a nightmare I can't wake up from," she added, saying that her son's death had also had a profound impact on her own mental health.[113]

Such things cannot be dismissed as 'something that doesn't happen here' and only relevant for emergency services and mental health units. The National Confidential Inquiry into Suicide and Homicide by People with Mental Illness (2014) showed that the majority of people are in contact with their GP prior to suicide.[114] Overall, 77% of individuals consult with their GP in the year before suicide, and 45% consult in the preceding month. Suicide risk increases with increasing number of GP consultations, particularly in the two to three months prior to suicide. In those who attended more than twenty-four times, risk was increased twelvefold. If a GP practice has not checked the premises for ligature points or other significant risks (such as access to a flat roof or unrestricted higher-floor windows) then there is likely to be a degree of censure if a patient leaves their consultation and attempts or completes suicide on the premises.

An NHS Trust was fined after a patient broke her spine falling from a first-floor window in 2011. The hospital was fined £10,000 by magistrates after admitting health and safety offences. The patient was in an apparent state of confusion when she used a chair to fully open a bay window and then climbed out. She fell onto bushes, which partly cushioned the fall, but had to be transferred for treatment to broken vertebrae and a punctured lung. Decent window restrictors, checked regularly and replaced if necessary, would probably have prevented the incident. There are numerous reported prosecutions where care home residents have fallen from unrestricted windows or windows with broken restrictors. The Commission dedicates a page of its website to the issue of falls from windows, and the HSE also offers guidance.[115,116]

---

113 Morrison S (2021) *Mental health trust fined £1.5m for failings over deaths of 11 patients* [online]. Available at: www.standard.co.uk/news/health/mental-health-trust-essex-fined-patient-deaths-b941038.html (accessed August 2023).

114 https://documents.manchester.ac.uk/display.aspx?DocID=37574 (accessed August 2023).

115 www.cqc.org.uk/guidance-providers/learning-safety-incidents/issue-7-falls-windows (accessed August 2023).

116 www.hse.gov.uk/healthservices/falls-windows.htm (accessed August 2023).

Key legislation

There are too many statutory requirements to cover in detail as part of this book. Large providers have whole teams dedicated to the oversight and maintenance of safe premises and equipment, and there is a requirement for registered managers to be aware of key legislation that impacts on their service. A systematic and logical approach to storage of evidence is essential if a 'Good' or better rating is wanted. Not all inspections will check everything – they cannot possibly do so, and some things will come up more regularly than others. Whether they are requested on inspection or not, providers need to ensure they can evidence compliance with the following (not intended as an exhaustive list):

- The Food Safety Act (1990)
- Fire Safety (England) Regulations 2022
- Gas Safety (Installation and Use) Regulations 1994
- The Health and Safety at Work Act (1974)
- Health and Safety Executive guidance such as that around Legionella and legionnaires' disease and electrical safety
- Health and Safety (Sharp Instruments in Healthcare) Regulations 2013
- Hazardous Waste (England and Wales) Regulations 2005
- The Controlled Waste Regulations 2012
- The Lifting Operations and Lifting Equipment Regulations 1998

In hospitals, the list is even longer and there are many specialist areas of environmental regulations to consider.

If a provider uses motor vehicles as part of their service provision, that adds to the regulatory burden. It is not just ambulance services that provide vehicles; care homes often have minibuses or cars, domiciliary care agency staff use cars, blood supply services use vehicles and so on. All need to be able to evidence that the equipment is safe, and to demonstrate safe practice in relation to the vehicles and drivers.

Evidence to support the Quality Statement

In terms of the different evidence sources around a safe environment and safe equipment, the documentary evidence is what is most likely to be reported on. While inspection teams will have conversations with staff and people using services, they are unlikely to be about the service environment or maintenance of equipment.

Evidence from data and records

What documentary evidence do you need and how can you ensure that you have all bases covered? The simple answer is to ensure that premises and equipment checks are carried out and recorded by someone who likes spreadsheets, governance and neat paperwork. In terms of Belbin's team roles, it needs a 'completer finisher' rather than a 'plant' or 'resource investigator'.[117] Belbin describes these people as being most effectively used at the end of tasks to polish the work and scrutinise it for errors, subjecting it to the highest standards of quality control. They are painstaking, anxious and conscientious. They search out errors, polishing and perfecting. Their insistence on detail and all the boxes being ticked may irritate occasionally, and they are easy to dismiss as blinkered and dull; they could even be accused of taking perfectionism to extremes. But they are exactly the people who are best at ensuring that there is evidence of compliance with the full range or relevant legislation.

I'd be hopeless at it; I would have lovely, neat spreadsheets for a few days or even weeks, and then go off on a tangent to some more exciting project. I score quite low on the completer finisher role – which is fine, as I'm aware of that and I can build a team where we have a completer finisher to ensure we deliver to expectations. Teams need different people in different roles, or they won't be effective. Registered managers are often not best placed to lead on estates and equipment governance. An innovative entrepreneur or charismatic, motivational leader often won't check that all the boxes are ticked. Leaders need to delegate to someone who likes detail and accuracy. Who enjoys audit and policy. And who likes being a bit of an expert on various pieces of legislation.

Getting the right person to delegate the oversight to is the most important step in maintaining and evidencing compliance. Giving them time and resources to do the job well is the second step. It might seem expensive to employ someone to do all the compliance checks, but it's much, much cheaper than a prosecution and much less painful for all involved than avoidable harm or an avoidable death. If care or clinical staff are not having to check the fire-safety systems or run off the water to prevent Legionella, then they have more time to focus on providing care. A multi-site provider can use the same person to cover several sites and maintain records across the group. A very large provider needs a team. The person who has the attention and focus to seemingly small things is a really valuable member of the team and should be treated as such; without them, censure is far more likely. What they do may well be seen as unimportant – until someone is injured or becomes very ill, and the provider is able to stand in a court with evidence that they had taken every step possible to reduce the risk of harm.

---

117 www.belbin.com/about/belbin-team-roles (accessed August 2023).

In fact, if the records are all completed as required, the provider is much less likely to find themselves in a court.

Many of the statutory premises and equipment safety checks can be contracted out, and they often are – for example, and most services will employ fire safety consultants to do all the fire safety work. That is good as such firms usually provide real expertise and ensure that the checks are timed to maintain compliance. They can offer fire risk assessments and staff training, extinguisher replacements and smoke detector checks. What they cannot do is take the responsibility for fire safety away from the provider or registered manager. That responsibility to provide safe care and treatment (Regulation 12) and to ensure that the regulated activities are delivered from safe premises, using safe equipment (Regulation 15) cannot be delegated. Providers can buy services such as fire safety equipment management, but they still need to maintain oversight of the contract and the way it is delivered. If fire doors which are meant to hold fire back for two hours are damaged and do not close properly, trapping people with a rapidly advancing fire, it will be the service provider who is prosecuted for failing to ensure compliance with the Fire Safety (England) Regulations 2022.

Having got a really good person to take responsibility, that person needs to be very clear about their remit, their responsibilities, the escalation processes and their route to raise concerns. It might be they have responsibility for fire safety, water safety, gas and electrical safety but not for maintenance of clinical equipment such as hoists or electrical bed and pressure-relieving mattresses. Alternatively, they might lead a team where one person manages oversight of waste management and food hygiene while another has a role focusing on security, environmental maintenance, odd jobs and a premises walk-around to check for trip hazards and other damage that could cause harm. It doesn't really matter what is or isn't included in their remit – what matters is clarity of expectations and an understanding of who does what.

The documentary evidence will need collating into accessible formats. Whether that is an inspector sitting with the head of estates looking at their electronic files, or reports submitted weekly to the registered manager confirming that the various checks have been completed and any issues identified (which are then filed in a designated file) is down to individual providers. What is important is that the provider and registered manager have assurance that the necessary checks are completed and that any shortcomings or risks are identified. There then needs to be a record showing that action was taken. That might be a RAG (Red, Amber, Green) checklist of weekly and daily tasks on a commercial database which are archived once all checks have been turned green and remedial actions taken, or it might be a manual maintenance logbook where staff write required jobs, and the estates person writes issues from their regular checks, and these are signed off once completed. The checks can be recorded using a diary, database or spreadsheet. It doesn't matter, as long as they are recorded and there is evidence that there is monitoring by the provider.

Everyday checks

That addresses the statutory checks and 'big estates' safety issues. There is still the bit about the everyday checks that staff usually have to do. These are the areas most commonly picked up on inspection, and which find their way into reports. They are not necessarily the things that will cause people the greatest harm, but they are often the focus of inspectors – I think because they are fairly easy to check and can be indicative of other issues. How do you make sure your drug-fridge temperature gets checked regularly? How do you make sure that staff record food holding and serving temperatures, or bathwater temperatures? How can you demonstrate that there is sufficient equipment for staff to do their jobs?

There are simple ways to ensure that equipment check records are complete. How providers choose to do this will depend on the size and nature of the service. The way to make sure it happens is to make it easy to achieve. Things to consider might be:

■ Automate the task. Invest in a temperature-monitoring system that sends alerts when there is a temperature outside the set parameters. This can be for drug storage or food holding and serving.

■ Make it a task for a named person. Ensure they know it is their responsibility and try to ensure it is done at a regular time, so that it is an embedded part of their routine. It doesn't have to be a Band 5 nurse who checks the drug-fridge temperatures or even the resuscitation equipment. There is nothing to stop a large provider such as an NHS Trust training a small group of volunteers to do it. Many early retired healthcare professionals might quite enjoy having a reason to be in a healthcare environment again. In smaller services, make it part of someone's job description – again, it doesn't have to be someone senior, it needs to be someone methodical and with attention to detail. That might be a receptionist in a GP practice, an administrator in a care home or a pharmacy assistant in an independent hospital. What matters is that they understand the task and why it is important, and that they have a route to escalate concerns. Obviously, that escalation route needs a means of recording not only what needed escalating, but the action required to put it right.

■ Block out dates when the service isn't providing care or treatment. Sometimes the gaps relate to days when the day surgery unit was closed or a ward in an independent hospital was not open. If the service is part-time, make sure the space to record daily checks is blocked out clearly so that there can be no assumption that checks were not carried out. Doing that ahead of closures means less time trying to work out why there were gaps in the record. If closures are due to resourcing and the last thing people are thinking about is filling in the drug-fridge temperature check form, then make sure the person responsible knows to clearly block out the preceding day or days when the unit was closed – this might be for a midwifery-led unit where staff were moved to ensure safe staffing on the main obstetric unit, or a single-handed dental practice where the dentist is too unwell to work for a few days.

■ Make it easy. Help people to do the right thing. Look at the systems you have in place for recording checks on premises and equipment. If you expect ambulance crews to walk back through three locked doors and use a computer to sign to say they have checked the ambulance stock before they go out on the road, then the signature is not very likely to appear, and even if they have checked there will be no record. Similarly, if the green 'I am clean' stickers are kept at the nurses' station rather than the dirty utility, they aren't going to be used very often. If the checklist is on paper in the ambulance and scanned onto the computer system each week (or put in a file in a records office) it is more likely to be completed. The alternative is to force people's hand. If the keys to an ambulance are not handed over until one of the crew swops them for a completed checklist, then the checklist will be completed and can be filed. Every service is different, and each provider must decide its own processes, but they should be mindful that the easier a process is to follow, the more likely it is to be followed.

■ Monitor compliance and act if essential checks are not being completed. That might be a ward sister or ward pharmacist checking the controlled drugs book each week and addressing any errors identified, or it might be a care home provider visiting the homes specifically to check that fire safety measures are being carried out in accordance with their policy. Both those monitoring processes should be recorded. Some larger providers can use their software programmes to provide evidence of monitoring. A provider of many care homes may use a system that allows them to show which staff were in which room at what time, how long call bells take to answer and daily maintenance checks. Most GP services and hospitals can monitor how long it takes for calls to be answered. A smaller provider will have to use more labour-intensive methods to audit practice. There are, to the best of my knowledge, no software systems that audit how often chaperones or interpreters are used or waiting times between checking in and being called to see a GP. Once again, how the monitoring is done is not important, but ensuring it is done and then used to make improvements is essential.

■ Have accessible records of checks and audits of checks. Store them where they can be found easily, even if the registered manager or whoever usually responds to a knock on the door by an inspection team is not around. Make sure key people know where records are. Too often (and more so for small providers or small locations) the inspection team ask for records of checks and incidents and get a blank stare from some poor junior member of staff who becomes increasingly stressed as the day progresses and can only shrug when asked for things. Some managers get too stressed to find things, too. Have everything stored in an easy-to-understand format in an accessible place – whether that be on a database or in paper format. If you have a bound notebook or loose-leaf file for incident recording, make sure there is a large label on the front that says 'Incident records'. In that file, keep the individual incident records (maybe a page for each report and response) and at the front have a separate page or pages that records incident report monitoring. Keep that file or book with the other records that would likely be required for inspection. If it's a computer-held record, make sure that there is always someone that can show the inspection team the records. If the registered manager is the only person with the password and they are on a three-week cruise around Japan, then there is likely to be a comment in any subsequent report that says incident records were requested but not available.

- Submit information that you were not able to provide, for whatever reason, on the day of an inspection. This is not about a risk to people using the service but a risk around the rating you are likely to get if information is not provided. If you have evidence that was not requested, or which was not found by the shift leader on the day, submit it via the portal as soon as possible afterwards with a note saying either it was not requested, or the member of staff wasn't sure where it was kept. If you supply the necessary information in the few days after an inspection, it must be considered, and the Commission cannot say there was no policy around premises security if you send a duly ratified and current policy two days after the inspection visit. It is perfectly reasonable that a flustered shift leader isn't sure where the policy is stored but knows there is one and what they need to do around security in their role.

- Similarly, use the factual accuracy process to provide additional evidence that for whatever reason was not shared on the day of the inspection nor requested afterwards. If a draft report says "Care staff said there were not enough staff to meet people's needs", provide records showing that staffing is planned and adjusted according to need, call-bell audits that show prompt answering of calls, monitoring of care records to ensure that care is delivered in line with plans, and feedback from service users, visitors and a staff survey that suggest otherwise. That is unless there really is a shortage, in which case accept the comment and adjust the staffing to better meet the needs of people using the service.

There also needs to be assurance around specialist equipment and staff that are not employed. This won't apply to all services, but a surprising number of services have specialist equipment that is either owned by the provider or, less usually, brought in by consultants. Not having ownership of, say, a laser used for ophthalmic surgery does not negate the provider from the need to have assurance about the safety of the machine and the environment within which it is used.

Evidence from staff and service users

As noted above, documentary evidence is paramount when considering the safety of a provider's service environment and equipment. Conversations with staff and people using services are not really likely to be about whether there is temperature monitoring of the holding temperature of the fish pie during lunch service.

Staff will, however, be asked whether they have enough equipment to do their jobs safely – and that will be service-type dependent. A care home won't need a resuscitaire (a device which combines a warming therapy platform along with the components needed for clinical emergency and resuscitation) to provide a warm surface on which to resuscitate and check newborns, but a maternity service will need to ensure they have sufficient for their busiest days and nights plus a few spare to allow for cleaning and maintenance.

An NHS Trust was inspected in January 2023 and the inspection team reported that:

"Equipment was not regularly serviced. We reviewed the equipment asset log and identified that a significant number were out of date for servicing. These included resuscitaires, LEDs for phototherapy, dopplers and fetal monitoring sonicaids. Information from the Trust showed a resuscitaire was due to be serviced on 29th April 2022 and this had not been serviced at the time of our inspection. The lack of appropriate monitoring of equipment exposed babies and mothers to the risk of harm as equipment may not be fit for use for routine care and in case of an emergency. During our review of information, we found an incident which occurred in July 2022, where a baby was born in an unexpectedly poor condition. The midwife-initiated resuscitation was ineffective due to appropriate equipment not being checked or available."[118]

Not only did the provider face regulatory action, but there was a real risk of poor outcomes for an infant and his or her family because of a lack of availability and poor governance of equipment.

---

118 CQC (2023) *William Harvey Hospital Inspection Report* [online]. Available at: https://api.cqc.org.uk/public/v1/reports/0cda8579-2699-4d08-8ada-285922c88341?20230616090943 (accessed August 2023).

Chapter 16: Safe and effective staffing

Quality Statement:

We make sure there are enough qualified, skilled and experienced people, who receive effective support, supervision and development. They work together effectively to provide safe care that meets people's individual needs.

Where do you even begin to know how many staff are needed for a service at any given time? The simple answer is that there is lots of guidance out there, along with several staffing-needs planning tools. That is true of many different services and in some cases, parts of services. There is staffing guidance from the Royal Colleges that not only gives the number of staff but also offers guidance around specific roles and the extent of cover required. The various guidance documents are readily available online, and they are the standards used when the Commission assesses staffing levels. NICE offer guidance on staffing in maternity units.[119] NHS England offers a more generic guide to nursing, midwifery and care staff requirements in healthcare settings.[120] Skills for Care offers guidance around staffing requirements in adult social care settings.[121] Some guidance, such as that issued by the Royal College of Anaesthetists, transfers across and is applicable to independent healthcare settings.[122]

The guidance is the starting point and a baseline for the minimum requirements in specific settings, but it does not usually offer specific numbers or a ratio of care workers to residents. That calculation has to be done by providers or registered managers (or those they delegate the task to), who must use the regulation as the basis for their calculations.

There are two key regulations relating to staffing requirements in registered services, Regulation 18: 'Staffing' and Regulation 19: 'Fit and proper persons employed', with a link to Regulation 12: 'Safe care and treatment'. That last regulation, Regulation 12, is how the provider should determine the staffing requirements for the regulated activities they provide and is also how compliance with Regulation 18 is judged. Quite simply, if care and treatment is provided in a safe way, with consideration of the individual needs and preferences of people using a service, then it is likely that there

---

119 www.nice.org.uk/guidance/ng4 (accessed August 2023).

120 www.england.nhs.uk/wp-content/uploads/2013/11/nqb-how-to-guid.pdf (accessed August 2023).

121 www.skillsforcare.org.uk/resources/documents/Support-for-leaders-and-managers/good-and-Outstanding-care/Improve-your-CQC-rating/Guide-to-safe-staffing.pdf (accessed August 2023).

122 www.rcoa.ac.uk/gpas/chapter-1 (accessed August 2023).

are sufficient staff – or, at least, it would be hard to argue that there are not. If, however, there are lots of medicines errors, if people are left in pain or are not supported to eat and drink enough, if people have lots of falls or develop pressure damage, and if the guidance around staffing is not adhered to, then it is likely that there are staffing shortfalls.

Regulation 19 is about employing fit and proper persons.[123] That does not mean people who can run marathons and who went to good schools. It means that persons employed for the purposes of carrying on a regulated activity must:

- Be of good character.
- Have the qualifications, competence, skills and experience which are necessary for the work to be performed by them.
- Be able by reason of their health, after reasonable adjustments are made, to properly perform tasks which are intrinsic to the work for which they are employed.

In order to maximise the chances of the people employed being 'fit and proper', recruitment procedures must be established and operated effectively. Regulation 19 requires that information about candidates set out in Schedule 3 of the regulations must be confirmed before they are employed. In a shortened form, it says that this means recruitment processes must include:

- A recent photograph.
- A DBS check at the level appropriate for the intended role.
- Evidence of suitable conduct in prior childcare, health or social care roles – usually references.
- The reason for leaving their previous childcare, health, or social care roles – usually a CV or employment history with gaps explained.
- Evidence of the person's qualifications – the original certificates are required.
- Validation of professional registration status.
- Details of any health condition or disability that might impact on their ability to carry out the role.

Selection and interview processes should assess the accuracy of applications and be designed to demonstrate candidates' suitability for the role, while meeting the requirements of the Equality Act (2010) in relation to pre-employment health checks. Recruitment checks on candidates may be carried out by a party other than the provider – in which case, providers must assure themselves that all checks are complete and satisfactory. If a

---

123 www.cqc.org.uk/guidance-providers/regulations-enforcement/regulation-19-fit-proper-persons-employed (accessed August 2023).

position requires someone to have a specific professional registration or the role requires use of a protected title, then the provider must ensure that the candidate has current registration and the necessary qualifications.

Where a person employed by the registered person no longer meets the criteria of a 'fit and proper' person, the provider must take appropriate action. If the person is a health care professional, social worker or other professional registered with a health care or social care regulator, they should inform the regulator in question.

Evidence to support the Quality Statement

As noted above, there are two key regulations relating to staffing requirements in registered services, Regulation 18: 'Staffing' and Regulation 19: 'Fit and proper persons employed'. I will look at each of this in turn, starting with Regulation 19.

Regulation 19: 'Fit and proper person employed'

Regulation 19: 'Fit and proper persons employed' is quite an easy regulation to demonstrate compliance with. Staff files need to be available with the required documentation. Larger providers will have their own human resources team or outsource recruitment, and only need to check once or twice a year that the process is being followed. Smaller providers are likely to do this for themselves, meaning that there is more scope to miss something – which is why there should be a recruitment policy and a recruitment checklist.

Most providers will need a checklist at the front of each file that shows what specific documentary evidence the recruitment process requires and confirmation that this has been supplied. That checklist should include the dates of the interview and whether an offer was made to the candidate. Behind the checklist should be a photocopy of qualifications certificates and professional registration certificates, plus evidence that ID has been checked to confirm the person is who they claim to be. This is usually a passport but could be a photocard driving licence.

Providers also need a system that reminds them to update staff files. Again, this is much easier for larger providers who have personnel databases and teams whose job is to manage workforce and record the checks. They still miss out key information, but less frequently than small providers do. It is easy to get caught out and not re-record that the six registered nurses employed all remain registered with the NMC. It is possible to leave the responsibility with the nurses to supply their updated registration date, but they might well forget. The system can be as simple as an entry in a diary (electronic or paper) each year to update the registration date of all staff with professional registration. In the same way, DBS check updates can be set as a reminder in a diary or electronic calendar. The length of time between checks should be detailed in the recruitment or safeguarding policies – but is usually three years.

There are times when some providers take shortcuts around recruitment or do not have records for individual staff members because of an existing relationship when the person is recruited. There is no exception in the regulation. This means if the nurse happens to be the provider's sister-in-law, the full recruitment process must still be followed. If the provider of a private skin clinic has worked alongside a dermatologist in an NHS hospital for year, the full recruitment process must still be followed. If the provider and another paramedic work together in an NHS Ambulance Trust and the other paramedic only does the odd shift, the full recruitment process must still be followed. A volunteer helping in a hospice library still requires a full recruitment process to be followed. The chef, the cleaner, the gardener, the activities co-ordinator, the chaplain – all require a full recruitment process. There are no exceptions.

Equality and discrimination

Regulation 19: 'Fit and proper persons employed' also requires providers to ensure that people employed are able by reason of their health, after reasonable adjustments are made, to properly perform tasks which are intrinsic to the work for which they are employed. That is harder to demonstrate and requires consideration of the Equality Act (2010) to make reasonable decisions. Employers must be mindful of the careful balancing act needed to ensure employees and potential employees are not discriminated against (both because a diverse workforce improves outcomes for people using services, increases innovation and widens the talent pool, and also because to do so would be to act unlawfully) and that staff provide safe, high-quality care to people using services. Every situation is different, and providers will need to make reasonable adaptations, where necessary, to enable staff with health challenges to remain in their workforce.

What holds true across all service types and with all grades of staff is that a provider cannot simply decide that someone cannot do a job because of physical or mental health limitations. Providers need to be able to demonstrate that they have sought expert advice from an occupational health consultant, and implemented the advice about what reasonable adaptations might enable an employee to continue to work.

As an example, a practice nurse who is an independent prescriber has a serious accident while cycling and becomes dependent on the use of crutches over short distances and a wheelchair for longer distances. The practice partners do not believe that the nurse can carry out his role and resort to unpleasant tactics to try and get him to realise this. They hold meetings upstairs when there are no lifts. They move the ground-floor staff room upstairs which means he cannot join others for lunch break. They remove the electric examination couch from the nurses' room and replace it with a standard high couch that he cannot reach. And the senior partner says that they are all doctors, and therefore they don't need an occupational health referral.

The partners in this case run the risk of losing a tribunal. It was high-risk for them to assume the nurse could not continue to work after the accident rather than seeking proper advice about how he could be supported to work. Some health conditions will indeed mean that a person is not safe to employ in specific roles and settings, but providers cannot just make arbitrary decisions about that. Someone living with bipolar disorder may have had suicidal thoughts or even attempted to end their life. They may not be suitable for employment in a pharmacy where there is ready access to powerful drugs, but that still needs employers to seek expert advice, to understand the impact of the condition on the employee and to determine whether reasonable adjustments could be made. A person may reasonably be barred from training to drive an ambulance if they had an epileptic seizure two years ago, but the provider still needs to seek the advice of the DVLA and occupational health to be on firm ground.

Is this issue one of safety, or one of employment rights and equality? I would argue that it is both. Clearly, someone who is so unwell they cannot carry out the work required of their role presents a risk to people using services; a paramedic who loses their sight cannot continue to drive, and a surgeon with frequent seizures despite medication cannot continue to perform neurosurgery. Both situations would be a clear safety risk for people using services. However, the health conditions described would not necessarily be barriers to all employment that uses the skills and experience of those individuals. And that is where it becomes an employment matter.

Regulation 18: 'Staffing'

The other key regulation with regard to this Quality Statement is Regulation 18: 'Staffing', which says that providers must deploy sufficient numbers of suitably qualified, competent, skilled and experienced persons in order to meet people's care and treatment needs. While shorter, this regulation is more open to interpretation and less specific in its guidance. It also tends to be where corners are cut in times of economic challenge, and that is very unwise as better staffing ratios reduce overall costs in most cases. While health care assistants may be cheaper on paper than registered nurses, there is good evidence that significant reductions in cost and length of stay may be possible with higher ratios of nurses in hospital settings. Sufficient numbers of registered nurses may prevent adverse events that cause patients to stay longer than necessary. Costs are also reduced with greater nurse staffing, as registered nurses have higher knowledge and skill levels to provide more effective nursing care, as well as to reduce patient resource consumption.[124]

Persons employed by a service provider in the provision of a regulated activity must receive such appropriate support, training, professional development, supervision and appraisal as is necessary to enable them to carry out the duties for which they are employed. They must also be enabled where relevant to obtain further qualifications appropriate to the work they perform. Where such persons are health care professionals, social workers or other professionals registered with a health or social care regulator, they must be enabled to provide evidence to the regulator in question demonstrating, where it is possible to do so, that they continue to meet the professional standards which are a condition of their ability to practise or a requirement of their role.

The most effective way to ensure on a continuous basis that there are sufficient staff, with the right qualifications and experience, to meet needs, is to monitor the quality of care and treatment being provided. The statutory guidance is intended to support providers in determining staffing models, but looking at outcomes for people using the service is a much clearer indication of when the balance of providing sufficient staff with an appropriate mix of skills against managing budgets is falling too heavily on the side of reduced costs and 'efficiency savings.' It might seem that you can simply replace GPs (who are hard to recruit and expensive to employ) with paramedics, physicians associates and pharmacists, but there is a risk to that.

Increasing the employment of staff with new clinical roles in primary care has been proposed as a solution to the shortages of GPs and nurses, and, increasingly, practices have a mixed workforce with representation of many healthcare disciplines. A study published in 2022 showed that increased numbers of GPs and nurses were positively associated with changes in practice activity and outcomes. Introducing new roles, however, was negatively associated with patient satisfaction; the study recognised that pharmacists improved prescribing practice but showed that all non-GP staff categories were associated with higher health system costs.[125] The authors highlighted that skill-mix changes increase capacity but also increase costs, reducing quality.

---

124 Thungjaroenkul P, Cummings GG & Embleton A (2007) The impact of nurse staffing on hospital costs and patient length of stay: a systematic review. *Nurs Econ*. Sep-Oct **25**(5): 255-65. PMID: 18080621.

125 Francetic I, Gibson J, Spooner S, Checkland K & Sutton M (2022) Skill-mix change and outcomes in primary care: Longitudinal analysis of general practices in England 2015–2019 [online]. Available at: www.sciencedirect.com/science/article/pii/S0277953622005305 (accessed August 2023).

Another study published in *The British Medical Journal* looked at the nursing workforce across Europe and concluded that, "A bedside care workforce with a greater proportion of professional nurses is associated with better outcomes for patients and nurses. Reducing nursing skill-mix by adding nursing associates and other categories of assistive nursing personnel without professional nurse qualifications may contribute to preventable deaths, erode quality and safety of hospital care and contribute to hospital nurse shortages."[126]

Clearly, then, effective staffing is not only about having more staff, but also about having better-qualified staff with the depth and breadth of underpinning knowledge to make safe decisions and to recognise deterioration or conditions that, if untreated, could increase avoidable mortality and worsen outcomes for people using services. Indeed, looking at outcomes and quality of care is a basic requirement when considering whether a staffing model is adequate, both in terms of numbers and in terms of skills and experience. A whiteboard showing that expected staffing was met on six out of seven days in the preceding week is only an indicator that the numbers of staff were usually as planned. That planning can be very variable, and it may not actually be as dynamic as needed to meet the needs of people on a hospital ward.

Assessing staffing requirements

Often, the best indicator of whether planned staffing numbers are adequate to meet patients' needs is to sit quietly in a corner somewhere, listen and watch. Such observation doesn't have to be done by the person planning the staffing numbers – although that can be a salutary learning experience. A volunteer or a peer ward manager can do it and fill in a report template that provides evidence of assessing staffing. Staff knowing that workloads and staffing are observed is a good thing – they need to know it is about workloads and staffing levels, rather than their own individual practice, but they will be delighted someone is trying to understand. If middle managers see firsthand what pressures staff are working under, then they may be more inclined to fight their corner a bit harder rather than applying more pressure.

A ward whiteboard may, and usually does, have the same numbers recorded as the planned level of staffing every day for five months. It is hard to imagine any real-life ward where the demands are so static, unless it is a highly specialist unit for eye surgery or long-term ventilated patients. Planning should be dynamic and reflect the needs of the patients being cared for on each shift. If the level of need increases because there are two patients approaching the end of their life and one patient who has been moved to the

---

126 Aiken LH, Sloane D & Griffiths P, for the RN4CAST Consortium et al (2017) Nursing skill mix in European hospitals: cross-sectional study of the association with mortality, patient ratings, and quality of care. *BMJ Quality & Safety.* **26** 559-568.

ward to free up a critical care bed, then the staffing level should be increased to allow the same quality of care to be provided. If the technical care needs are such that the patients need the input of a registered nurse (perhaps because of their needs after leaving a critical care unit) then offering an additional healthcare assistant will not be sufficient.

In care homes or independent hospitals, similar observations can be carried out to understand the quality of care and how staffing levels affect this. The record of these observations is evidence of monitoring of staffing. Some providers invest in electronic monitoring systems which show the provider, or the registered manager, how quickly call bells are answered and where staff have been to check on people who have chosen to remain in their own rooms. The reports should be an add-on to direct observations of staff workload.

Sitting in a corner of the dining room watching how long people have to wait between mouthfuls, how long they sit at a table waiting for lunch and how many people each member of staff is supporting to eat or drink is a good way to assess whether staffing levels are sufficient at mealtimes. The provider may determine that staffing needs to be increased at lunchtime to reduce the need for people to sit for an hour at a dining table while others are helped to their seats, or for a care assistant to support three people to eat at the same time (thus increasing risk). There may be a primary school in the next road, with a parent who is delighted to have the chance to work from midday until three, five days a week, then scoot off to pick up the children. Not only does that solve the problem of lunchtime support, it also has long-term potential if that parent wants more hours as their children reach secondary school age. Wins all round!

Thinking about when additional staff are needed, and what they are needed for, will help providers to decide what job to offer, the hours, the role and where best to recruit. Thinking flexibly about that, rather than simply assuming that someone must work thirty-seven hours over five days with alternating late and early shifts, may prevent unnecessarily limiting ways of working and enable more creative solutions.

Contingency planning

Every provider needs a backup plan in case staff shortages occur for any reason. Smaller and more specialist services requiring staff with specific qualifications have less flexibility, and thus an even greater need for this. Whatever the service, it is not possible to just call the mother-in-law and ask if she is busy (unless she has been recruited properly and is a legitimate member of the bank staff). Reducing staff attrition and sickness goes a long way to reducing the need for staff at short notice – and that process is cyclical. Lower staff turnover and absence means less stress for everyone, which means that staff are more likely to turn up regularly and not leave to work for better-staffed providers. Even with low turnover and sickness rates, though, there will still be times when a backup plan is needed.

In some services, the backup plan might mean closing the service for a while. If one dentist from a two-dentist partnership injures their hand rock-climbing, then the practice needs to call patients, apologise, and tell them that they need to rearrange their appointments. The remaining dentist might be able to squeeze in an extra patient or two, but they will be sufficiently stretched with their own list and emergencies so that probably isn't sustainable for more than a few days and the injured dentist's list will need to be cancelled.

If a care home has an outbreak of norovirus that affects several staff members, they cannot simply close the doors and an alternative solution needs to be sorted so that care continues to be provided to a high standard. That might mean some staff doing overtime, or it might mean using bank or agency staff. If there is more than one home in close proximity to others in the same ownership, there are benefits to ensuring contracts and usual practice are the same so that staff can work in different homes. Each of three homes having one less member of staff per shift for three days is far better than one home having three fewer staff. Staff rotating between homes also encourages sharing of best practice, offers greater scope for development and reduces the risk of a closed culture developing. Staff want to build a sense of ownership of their service and create a cohesive team, but safety across the provider group is the priority in the event of an unplanned staffing crisis. If staff have to be moved at short notice frequently, there is probably a lesson to be learned about safe staffing levels.

However providers address staffing shortfalls and the need for contingency plans, they still need to be assured and to be able to evidence that the people providing care are 'fit and proper'. That means they must be recruited and trained for the role being asked of them. A midwifery postnatal ward where there is a significant unpredicted staffing shortfall might reasonably ask a registered nurse to cover for one absent midwife, as there are many tasks with which the nurse could support the established ward staff (although there must still be midwives deployed). However, it would be entirely inappropriate to staff a delivery suite entirely with registered nurses, and the provider would need to have plans to find sufficient midwives to provide safe care to birthing mothers and their babies.

What providers should *not* do is wait until there is a staffing crisis and then scrabble around hoping to find someone to cover. There must be a protocol that is clear about what the plans are, including when and how they would be implemented. The wise provider will be overly generous in their contingency planning, and not just have minimal arrangements – if one staff member is off with norovirus, then the law of averages suggest that more will follow. Planning ahead for shortfalls is the best way to ensure continuity of sufficient staff to deliver high-quality care.

Chapter 17: Infection prevention and control

Quality Statement:

We assess and manage the risk of infection. We detect and control the risk of it spreading and share any concerns with appropriate agencies promptly.

This Quality Statement should, in theory, be an easy thing for any service to say with hand on heart. All services should be assessing and managing risks associated with infection – and in fairness most do a pretty good job, but many still get caught out by missing simple things. That is usually providers or managers not seeing what is in front of them, and that's why objective observation and fresh eyes are so important. Walk-arounds by a third party are a bit of a golden thread, and they really are invaluable – as long as they are structured and offer more than a nice chat with a few friendly-looking staff and service users.

The starting point for any infection prevention and control (IPC) strategy is a policy based on the national guidance and current best practice. COVID has certainly brought the need for good infection prevention and control measures to the forefront of everyone's consciousness, but the need has always been there, and it will continue long after we have stopped seeing 'Hands, Face, Space' slogans peeling off walls around every corner. In the flu season of 2022-23, nearly 15,000 excess deaths associated with influenza were reported. This was the highest figure since the 2017-18 season, which had 22,500 excess deaths.[127] During the COVID pandemic, the incidence of influenza reported to the WHO from across the world fell significantly. Epidemiologists believe that this is due to the public health measures taken by governments and health agencies to stop the spread of COVID, which also stopped influenza. These measures varied from country to country, but usually included isolation, mask-wearing and social distancing.

That reduction in the spread of influenza was made possible by good infection prevention and control measures. Interestingly, but unsurprisingly, other viral illnesses also reduced throughout the pandemic. Children were not mixing as much so cases of chicken pox reduced, teenagers were not able to do what teenagers often do so laryngitis, tonsillitis and glandular fever incidence reduced. Of real economic

---

127 Mahase E (2023) Flu deaths in the UK hit five year high last winter. *BMJ* 381. Available at: www.bmj.com/content/381/bmj.p1445 (accessed August 2023).

importance to providers is that, from March 2020, there was a decline in the number of reports of norovirus recorded by England's national laboratory surveillance system.[128] I don't think anyone would want such restrictive measures reinstated, and the financial cost is not the only consideration when thinking about how rigorous infection prevention and control measures should be, but the figures do demonstrate the scale of the problem, the resources that could be used in other ways and how effective at reducing costs and improving outcomes good infection prevention and control measures are.

Infection prevention and control has quite a small mention in the regulations. Regulation 12: 'Safe care and treatment' says simply that providers and registered managers must ensure that care and treatment is provided in a safe way for service users by "assessing the risk of, and preventing, detecting and controlling the spread of, infections, including those that are health care associated." The guidance about this part of Regulation 12 is not lengthy either:

"The Department of Health has issued a Code of Practice about the prevention and control of healthcare associated infections Health and Social Care Act 2008: Code of Practice on the prevention and control of infections and related guidance. The law says that CQC must take the Code into account when making decisions about registration and by any court during legal proceedings about registration. By following the Code, providers will be able to show how they meet this regulation, but they do not have to comply with the Code by law. A provider may be able to demonstrate that they meet this regulation in a different way (equivalent or better) from that described in the Code."[129]

That doesn't mean that the Code of Practice can be glanced at and dismissed knowing that there is hand gel in the reception area and a cleaner comes in after work each day. It needs to be studied and considered when thinking about infection prevention and control in each location. The document is the 'Health and Social Care Act 2008: Code of practice on the prevention and control of infections and related guidance'.[130] The comment about not having to comply with the Code by law does not actually mean that providers do not have to comply with it.

---

128 Ondrikova N *et al* (2021) Differential impact of the COVID-19 pandemic on laboratory reporting of norovirus and Campylobacter in England: A modelling approach. *PLoS One*. 2021 Aug 25;16(8). Available at: https://pubmed.ncbi.nlm.nih.gov/34432849/ (accessed August 2023)

129 CQC (2023) *Regulation 12: Safe care and treatment* [online]. Available at: www.cqc.org.uk/guidance-providers/regulations-enforcement/regulation-12-safe-care-treatment (accessed August 2023).

130 Gov.uk (2022) *Health and Social Care Act 2008: code of practice on the prevention and control of infections* [online]. Available at: www.gov.uk/government/publications/the-health-and-social-care-act-2008-code-of-practice-on-the-prevention-and-control-of-infections-and-related-guidance/health-and-social-care-act-2008-code-of-practice-on-the-prevention-and-control-of-infections-and-related-guidance (accessed August 2023).

It simply means that the Code was issued as guidance, is not a statutory instrument and cannot be enforced as something that legally must happen. The reality is that the Commission will use the Code of Practice to pin various observed or data deficiencies in care and treatment delivery to, and the enforcement would be against Regulation 12.

Transmission risk and isolation

Criterion 5 of the Code of Practice is that there is a policy for ensuring that people who have or are at risk of developing an infection are identified promptly and receive the appropriate treatment and care to reduce the risk of transmission of infection to other people. That is something all providers need to be able to demonstrate and explain to an inspection team. Clearly, the reason for the criterion is to reduce the risk of the spread of infection and serious consequences of an untreated infection. What that policy says and requires of staff will differ by type of service and the needs of the people using it. A sexual health clinic is unlikely to need to isolate someone with gonorrhoea, but an acute hospital in an area with an international airport and flights arriving from Madagascar or other areas of Africa might need to ensure they have facilities to isolate patients with suspected or confirmed tuberculosis in a negative pressure isolation room, (or an isolation room with a positive pressure ventilated lobby).

Care home providers and managers rarely need separate isolation facilities, as most people have individual bedrooms, and they usually have ensuite facilities. The policy would simply need to say that people will be isolated in their rooms, with heightened infection, prevention and control measures, until the risk of transmission to others has passed. They aren't likely to be caring for people with plague, but norovirus spreads very quickly and strict isolation and stringent preventative measures will reduce the risk of more people becoming ill.

What about other types of services? A GP practice needs to be ready for whatever walks through the door – even a child with suspected chicken pox or rubella will pose a risk to others who are immunosuppressed, or who are newly pregnant but unvaccinated. There needs to be somewhere that such a child can wait until they are seen, or some other way of avoiding people who are vulnerable to harm from contact with the infection. Seating them in different areas of the waiting room isn't sufficient. Receptionists must have a clear policy about who, when and how to ensure that patients are isolated if they pose a risk to others. If physical isolation isn't possible, an alternative can be isolation by timing – maybe have the child come in for the last appointment of a list, after everyone else has been seen and has left the premises.

An emergency ambulance crew are unlikely to be carrying more than one person at a time, but they still need a clear policy from their provider about the action to take if they respond to a call where there is clearly an infection transmission risk that requires isolation. If they arrive at an airport and collect a very unwell person with a high temperature, they need to have serious infections ruled out before leaving them on a trolley in the majors area of a busy accident and emergency department. The ambulance is a very effective isolation room until proven otherwise in this situation.

Translating guidance into practice

There are ten criteria at the start of the Code. Providers need to consider how their service will meet each standard and ensure that their own policies and guidance documents are aligned with the requirements.

Some of the guidance in the Code overlaps with other Quality Statements, and there may well be overlapping policies and evidence. The second criterion is about the provision and maintenance of a clean and appropriate environment in managed premises that facilitates the prevention and control of infections. This may be partially covered in the Quality Statement about safe environments, but it still needs to be covered in the infection prevention and control policy and practice. Running off the water delivery outlets that are not used very often, to reduce the risk of Legionella, is probably a task of maintenance staff – but oversight needs to be maintained by those responsible for infection prevention and control, and the policy needs to cover what happens if anyone develops Legionella-type symptoms.

Usually, expert advice is needed to ensure that an infection prevention and control policy is a useful document for the service it applies to. Fortunately, expert advice is quite readily available for most services. Many providers in a local Integrated Care System will be able to access the resources and expertise of an infection prevention and control team, and they should make use of that to ensure they are delivering best practice. The system infection prevention and control leaders may well have policies that can be adapted to each setting, and which ensure that providers are working collaboratively to the same standards and pathways. It is in everyone's best interests that care home providers and domiciliary care agencies have very good infection prevention and control practices, as it reduces the burden of unwell people needing ambulances, GP care and acute hospital care.

Evidence to support the Quality Statement

As noted at the beginning of this chapter, the starting point for any effective IPC strategy is a policy based on national guidance and current best practice. Beyond that, the single most powerful thing a service can do is to initiate walk-arounds by a third party with fresh eyes to check that simple things are not being missed.

Evidence from data and records

In terms of the documentary evidence regarding this Quality Statement, what is needed to demonstrate compliance? A current policy, obviously, that aligns with current best practice, national guidance and the Code, is reviewed and ratified, and is accessible and known to staff. Then, whatever documents there are that evidence that the policy is properly implemented and monitored, and which support the claim that the service is mindful of the importance of infection prevention and control.

- Staff-training records for all staff. Cleaners and caterers need infection prevention and control (IPC) training as much as nurses. The training might be different but handwashing, use of PPE, waste disposal and good personal hygiene are essential for all. Food-hygiene training is also needed for many roles.

- Cleaning schedules that show staff who do the cleaning what they should actually be cleaning, when and how. That might be a simple checklist of how to clean an ambulance at the end of a shift, or it might be a more complex kitchen-cleaning schedule broken down into daily, weekly and deep-clean tasks. There needs to be a record showing that regular cleaning tasks have been completed.

- Many places use green 'I am clean' stickers as a way of demonstrating that equipment is cleaned each time it is used. They are not mandated, but they are a good way to evidence this – if used properly. Too often, they simply show that staff have run out of stickers and have not had time to go to the ward store cupboard for more. If stickers are used, then they should be used diligently.

- Walk-around records. Walk-arounds can be done by a peer reviewer, an IPC lead or team member, a non-executive director, a student, a Healthwatch volunteer, a paid consultant or an independent person – any of whom can make a relatively unannounced tour of the premises with fresh eyes. Is there sufficient PPE available? Are staff using it and do they wash their hands? Does the place look clean and tidy? What does it smell like? What does the sluice/dirty utility look like? Are fridges clean? Are lavatories clean? What about showers and baths?

Choose someone fastidious who would prefer a high-class hotel to camping, who brings a napkin with their packed lunch, who is *really* fussy. These are the people who will spot the grimy plughole and the mildew on a shower curtain.

■ Audits. Good infection prevention and control requires monitoring. It is very easy for things to be overlooked at busy times – for missed checks to be normalised and seen as unimportant. My experience is that inspection teams always pick up on things that are easy to spot, and the degree of risk from an incomplete task may not necessarily be the thing that individuals focus on. While we should all focus on outcomes for people using services, it is much easier to fill a report with hard data that shows that there were two pieces of equipment (a commode and a shower chair, for example) that did not have 'I am clean' stickers, in line with policy.

Audits and assessments

Picking a few reports at random, a theme that comes up time and time again with regard to infection prevention and control – and which almost invariably leads to lowered ratings – is audits and governance. In May 2023, a care home report said, "Building related risks had not been well managed. A legionella risk assessment had not been carried out. The provider had not ensured that water flushing of unused outlets were being completed weekly. This meant the provider could not be assured that hot and cold-water outlets were at safe temperatures. Cold-water outlets being too warm can cause the growth of legionella bacteria. This put people at risk of harm."

In the same month, another care home report said, "The premises were not always clean. We saw that some communal areas, including dining rooms and bathrooms, were dirty and had not been effectively cleaned. This meant people's living environment was not always clean or suitable for use. Equipment was not always clean or properly maintained. For example, tables and chairs in dining areas were stained and dirty. Some shower chairs were also stained with dirt. Infection prevention and control systems were not always effective. For example, clinical waste was not always disposed of correctly and in line with the provider's policy. We also saw that personal protective equipment was not stored correctly to ensure it was free from contamination. The premises were not always clean or well-maintained. This was a breach of Regulation 12(1) of the Health and Social Care Act 2008 (Regulated Activities) Regulations 2014."

In the case of the second home, better monitoring and audits would have highlighted the concerns, and fresh-eyes walk-arounds would probably have prevented the lowered rating and enforcement action. Every provider should have an audit plan, and it needs to be followed. It is no use if a matron says they were too busy and just haven't had a chance to check whether the equipment was clean. I wouldn't sit on a soiled lavatory seat, and nobody else should have to. If the person responsible is too busy, then the task should be delegated – a master's degree in nursing is not necessary to spot that there are no 'I am clean' stickers on commodes, or that there are faeces smeared down a wall.

As ever, different service types will need different monitoring audits – although handwashing audits should be universal, and there should be clear evidence of action if compliance rates are low. Likewise, anywhere where people sleep on beds should have mattress and pillow audits, to check that underneath the covers the mattress is not wet, stained, or soiled. If it is, it needs replacing. Similarly, if pillows are not wipeable, they must be hygienic. I am sure most people pull the sheets off hotel beds to check the state of the mattress; in the same way, people in premises providing health or social care need to know that their pillows and beds are clean.

NHS services need to complete audits against the National Standards of Healthcare Cleanliness 2021.[131] The guidance from NHS England is comprehensive and includes audit arrangements. Large social care providers might want to read the guidance too and possibly adapt it for their services. Conversely, specialist services need audits of cleaning and decontamination of their specialist equipment against the manufacturer's guidance or their own policies. That might be cleaning operating theatre equipment, ventilator cleaning in a critical care unit or vehicle cleaning in an ambulance service.

Audits don't have to be overly burdensome or complex. Simple visual checks sometimes suffice – the external waste-storage facility is a case in point. This is often overlooked, but services are required to have a secure and safe environment for the storage of potentially hazardous waste. It really doesn't take an inspection team member very long to walk outside, see an overflowing skip with a mixture of orange, yellow and purple sacks, some which have fallen to the ground and been torn or ripped open, revealing contaminated material strewn around. In the same way, it doesn't take a member of staff or a provider very long to do the same.

Infection data and evidence of responses to data suggestive of worsening outcomes

This applies to independent hospitals and acute NHS hospitals particularly, but care homes need to monitor infection rates and outbreaks across their provider group or compared to other local providers (via the Integrated Care System), and GP practices need to look at the data around their

---

131 www.england.nhs.uk/wp-content/uploads/2021/04/B0271-national-standards-of-healthcare-cleanliness-2021.pdf (accessed August 2023).

management of infection and their prescribing practice. The Royal College of General Practitioners offers a range of audit templates that have been developed by NICE.[132] Ambulance Trusts probably won't have infection rates but should still be looking at outcome data for patients where there is a delayed response to concerns around infections, and where patients have not been taken to hospital and have suffered harm related to this, including undiagnosed serious infections. If the outcomes are assessed against protected characteristics, so much the better, and this is a good way to review how health inequalities are being reduced within the provider service and the local Integrated Care System.

Evidence from staff and service users

Evidence from service users

When an inspection team visits, team members should talk to people using the service. Usually, if the documentary evidence is available and is an honest account of the effectiveness of the infection prevention and control measures, people will be able to talk about them. People using the service might be asked whether their room or the ward bay is cleaned regularly and whether the bathrooms and lavatories are clean. They might be asked about staff washing their hands or other IPC measures such as PPE when providing care. They won't be asked about antibiotic stewardship or surgical site infections. Providers cannot coach people using the service to say the right thing – but then if providers do the right thing, people will say this anyway.

Evidence from staff

What staff are asked will depend on the type of service and the grade the staff member is working at. A Chief Nurse who is also the Director of Infection Prevention and Control would be expected to have a far better grip on the data, the strengths and challenges around infection prevention and control than a healthcare assistant in the outpatient department.[133] A pharmacist will be asked more about antibiotic stewardship than a care home cook, but the care home cook will likely be asked more about food-hygiene measures. When inspecting the end-of-life care core service in acute settings, mortuary staff are more likely to be asked about infection prevention and control measures than a specialist palliative medicines consultant or the chaplain.

---

132 https://elearning.rcgp.org.uk/mod/book/view.php?id = 12649 (accessed August 2023).

133 A Director of Infection Prevention and Control (DIPC) is a role required by all registered NHS care providers with the requirements detailed in the Code of Practice.

It isn't hard to work out the type of things staff will be asked about if the tasks associated with the highest risks of infection transmission are considered. As part of their ongoing development and supervision, it would be usual to have discussions with staff around their own infection prevention and control measures and how they meet the policy requirements in their work. If there are incidents related to infection transmission, such as a norovirus or Campylobacter outbreak, there should be a discussion and learning from that incident – and so staff would be indirectly prepared for inspection questions. If a GP practice was an outlier in antibiotic prescribing, one hopes that there would be a review of why that might be and whether there was any action or learning needed to address overprescribing. As part of usual good leadership practice, managers and leaders should be addressing infection prevention and control practice and knowledge, challenging poor practice, and not turning a blind eye because it is easier than asking someone with twenty years' experience to clean away their mess or to tell a nurse who vomited earlier in the day to go home despite staff shortages.

Staff don't need specific coaching on the perfect answer – there should be no need if practice is good. Practice should be good. They might, however, need coaching to give those answers and to have their anxieties allayed, so practising questions in team meetings might help them feel more comfortable with questions on inspection. They might need a phrase and permission to explain that they are feeling really stressed about the inspection and are too flustered to think of an example now, but that they will go away, think and come back with the answer to a specific question.

Proportionality and right to challenge

Infection prevention and control is one area where, I believe, it is sometimes reasonable to challenge an inspection report on grounds of proportionality. Nobody wants dirty premises or equipment, and nobody wants soiled bedding or staff with body odour, but for larger services the narrative in a report can sometimes be presented as the norm rather than something that is not statistically significant. Challenge is offered at the factual accuracy response stage and should be used where there is evidence that the report is not an accurate reflection of the service.[134]

I wouldn't encourage everyone to challenge, as most of the narrative and ratings are a fair reflection of what was found and what the evidence shows. However, if there is evidence that shows the narrative about what staff say, or an observed element of care (such as people being supported

---

134 For more about factual accuracy checks, see www.cqc.org.uk/factualaccuracyform-appendix (accessed August 2023).

with handwashing before meals), is not reflective of usual practice, then providers owe it to their staff to present that evidence and ask for the report to be amended. The factual accuracy process is not just about infection prevention and control, so the idea of challenge can be thought about for other aspects of a report. What is important is that, whatever the challenge, it must be evidenced.

In 2018, an acute NHS hospital was rated as 'Requires Improvement' for a number of reasons, including the following:

- "We observed three members of staff that were not compliant with the uniform policy.
- Curtains around beds on the ward were not disposable and did not have dates displayed so it was not possible to tell if they had been changed in line with infection control requirements."

The hospital in question employs more than four thousand staff. That is 0.075%; not exactly statistically significant when one thinks that significance is typically set to 0.05 or 5%. This means the inspection team were judging the hospital staff's compliance on the behaviour of a tiny proportion of staff, and that the judgement was therefore probably invalid. It remained in the published report, so I do not know whether there was a challenge or not. The narrative did not say that this suggested a wider attitude to compliance with the uniform policy, but it was in the report, which is about the provider rather than the individual staff members, so the evidence should be about the provider. If the provider had any audits that showed good compliance with uniform requirements and dress codes, and staff or team meeting records that showed that poor compliance with the uniform policy was addressed, then it would be reasonable to challenge the 'we saw three staff' as not being proportionate.

Similarly, the second part of the report quoted was about not having dates on curtains – a similar issue to green 'I am clean' stickers. I am sure the team did see curtains without a date displayed. What the report does not say is what infection prevention and control requirements they are referring to. The guidance simply requires that curtains/blinds should be visibly clean with no blood or body substances, dust, dirt, debris, stains or spillages. The CQC guidance acknowledges guidelines by the Infection Control Nurses Association which state there should be a procedure in place for regular decontamination of curtains.[135] There was no suggestion that the curtains appeared dirty, so there was probably scope for challenge if there was documented evidence around how the person responsible for changing curtains knew when to change them. That would, however, require more

---

135 See www.mysurgerywebsite.co.uk/website/IGP367/files/CQC_Guidance_Curtains-Sept2014.pdf (accessed August 2023).

than a note on a factual accuracy response saying, "Gaynor in estates is a real whizz and remembers everything!" It would require a policy that stated the expected frequency of curtain changes, along with written evidence of the last change and the planned date to change them again.

It might be worth remembering that there is no need to have a sticker or date to be written in semi-permanent ink on the hem of curtains. It's quite likely that busy ward staff (in this case, midwives on a maternity unit) would not know when curtains were changed and who did it. Why would they need that specific knowledge to care for women in labour? That evidence might be in A4 diary belonging to Gaynor in estates with an entry that said, 'maternity unit, children's ward, cardiology and haematology ward curtains change due on 14 April 2018' with a big tick to show it was completed and a further entry that said, 'maternity unit, children's ward, cardiology and haematology ward curtains change due on 12 October 2018' (a few months after the inspection date). It might be an electronic diary entry, or it might be a wall chart used for scheduling. The system doesn't matter – if, after reading the draft report, the provider knows they have evidence that challenges the comments in the report, they should share it with the Commission and ask that the report be amended.

That's the point of the factual accuracy – there should be recognition and agreement on the part of both the Commission staff and the provider that the report is accurate and a fair representation of the service.

Chapter 18: Medicines optimisation

Quality Statement:

We make sure that medicines and treatments are safe and meet people's needs, capacities and preferences by enabling them to be involved in planning, including when changes happen.

This is probably the Quality Statement that most providers would feel they met well and could say with confidence that they were compliant with. Certainly, the guidance and legislation around medicines management is very clear – although it should be added that optimisation is a step on from management.

Each year in England there are around 237 million errors in the medication process; 66 million of these are clinically significant, with the rest resulting in no or low harm. Avoidable drug errors are estimated to cost the NHS around £98.5 million a year, taking up 181,626 bed-days, as well as contributing to 1,708 deaths.[136] That is an awful lot of medication errors and potential for unsafe care and treatment. A 2021 Department of Health funded project on medication safety in care homes showed that on any one day, seven out of ten patients experienced at least one medication error. While the potential of most errors to cause harm was relatively low, the results did indicate an opportunity for more serious harm.[137]

This is an area of the regulatory framework where the Commission has its own specialist inspectors with a professional background in pharmacy. That's a good thing for people using services, as shortcomings will be picked up and measures taken to ensure that improvements make medicines safe for people using services. The Commission pharmacy team are real experts in the safe management of medicines. For providers, that means that they can't get around the need for safe systems or hope the inspection team won't notice a few mistakes – they will. That said, the pharmacy specialists don't necessarily attend all inspections, but providers should provide care and treatment knowing that a pharmacist might be part of the team, particularly if there have been any concerns around medicines optimisation.

---

136 Elliot RA, Camacho E & Jankovic D (2021) Economic analysis of the prevalence and clinical and economic burden of medication error in England. *BMJ Qual Saf* **30** (2) 96-105.

137 National Care Forum (2021) *Medication safety in care homes* [online]. Available at: www.nationalcareforum.org.uk/wp-content/uploads/2019/11/Medication-safety-project-summary-report.pdf (accessed August 2023).

This Quality Statement is about more than simply ensuring that controlled drugs books are accurately completed and that medication records are filled in accurately. It encompasses consent, which requires a default position that most people can decide whether to take their prescribed medicine and are entitled to information to help them make decisions around the medication being suggested or offered. Some providers need to consider covert administration, while others will need to consider when to stop administering drugs as someone's life draws to a close. The Quality Statement covers governance and the medication supply and disposal chains, along with safe storage and administration. It also covers antibiotic stewardship, vaccination programmes, unlicenced drugs and drug interaction risks. It is a huge area, but there is already good practice and plenty of guidance available.

It is very easy to dismiss medication errors as the human failings of an individual – indeed many, many incident reports do exactly that. Much more often, though, the true root causes are multifactorial. Improving medication safety is a systems issue. Most catastrophic errors are caused by a series of small errors which, individually, may have a low risk of harm but together present significant risks.

An example – prescription error

In 2015, a junior doctor was permanently removed from the General Medical Council register after a patient died of poisoning. The doctor had written milligrams instead of micrograms on a prescription while the patient was being treated at their local hospital. The patient had mental health problems and was detained in 2010 (it takes a long time for a case to reach a hearing). The patient fell and broke their hip while detained and was transferred to the local hospital where they had surgery. During the post-operative period, the patient was found to have an irregular heartbeat along with a couple of other problems. The doctor should have prescribed 250 micrograms of digoxin, a drug which regulates the heart, but wrote milligrams instead. It was later found that five 500-microgram containers of digoxin had been used; equivalent to a thousand times the intended dose. The patient had a heart attack and sadly could not be revived.

The doctor was struck off not only for the one incident, but also for several incidents and behaviours that fell short of those expected by the GMC. The incident is the focus here, though. How did that happen? Was it all down to one junior doctor? Were there things that others could have done to prevent it happening? It was a reaction to an urgent condition, so the prescription lacked the oversight from a pharmacist that would usually happen, but one imagines that the junior doctor did not go to the drug cupboard and administer the drug without a nurse being present, or even assisting. Certainly, if the drugs were obtained from the resuscitation trolley, someone else would have been supporting the doctor. It would be very odd for ward staff to see a doctor take drugs from the tamper-proof drawer of a trolley and not ask what was happening.

What other factors were there that compounded the problem? The doctor was said to be wilfully neglectful, but could a nurse pointing out that using five large phials of digoxin is unusual and perhaps they should check the dosage have prevented the mistake? There is no suggestion it was a deliberate attempt to harm, but rather that it was carelessness (and in fairness, the Trust reported to the GMC because of a series of careless mistakes rather than a single error). The patient was on an orthopaedic ward where the use of digoxin by intravenous injection would not be the norm – is there something about healthcare professionals responding to conditions they are not familiar with? The maximum emergency loading dose for an adult in atrial fibrillation is 0.75-1 mg, to be given over at least two hours according to the British National Formulary; is there something about the amount of stock drugs that should be held in one location and the risk assessments around this? Mistakes and incidents should lead to questions, and each question should be answered when an investigation is required. Not asking questions as part of a review of an incident risks repetition.

Accountability

The Commission does prosecute for medicines management failings. It does not regulate individual practitioners, so providers and registered managers who dismiss all medicines errors as being about a lack of competency, distraction, human failing, neglect or intent of individuals without considering the wider medicines pathway and their organisation's responsibilities may find they are being held to account.

In 2018, a care home provider and a registered manager were prosecuted, and each received a £4,000 fine.[138] A frail and vulnerable resident moved into the home for respite care. They arrived at the home with a bag of medicines including painkillers. The same day, the GP provided the home with details of the medicines prescribed to the resident. The provider and registered manager failed to check what prescribed medicines the resident should have been taking. Their systems failed to identify that those medicines had been incorrectly transcribed onto the resident's medicine administration record, which led to them failing to identify that too many painkillers had been written down. They then failed to check that staff followed their medicines policy. Five days after moving to the home, the resident died of an overdose of painkillers.

---

138 CQC (2022) *Medicines management – assessment* [online]. Available at: www.cqc.org.uk/guidance-providers/learning-safety-incidents/issue-9-medicines-management (accessed August 2023).

The Commission found unsafe medicines practices at the home, including:

- No assessment carried out, including medication needs.
- No care plan written about what care and support was needed.
- Failure to check what was currently prescribed.
- Incorrectly transcribing medicines to the medicine administration record.
- Incorrectly recording medicine to be taken regularly rather than PRN (pro re nata, meaning as and when required).
- Failure to record variable doses administered (one or two tablets).
- Painkillers being given when the resident was not in pain.
- Having only one staff member booking medicines in, when two were required.
- Lack of oversight and checks of the medicines being administered.

In the same year, the then-Health Secretary, Jeremy Hunt, voiced concerns about the scale of drug errors that were occurring. The numbers are above but it bears repeating that GPs, pharmacists, hospitals and care homes are estimated to be making 237 million errors a year – the equivalent of one mistake made for every five drugs handed out. A fifth of the mistakes in the study related to hospital care, including errors made by doctors administering anaesthetic before surgery.[139] The rest were pretty evenly split between drugs given in the community by GPs and pharmacists, and those handed out in care homes. There is plenty of guidance available from professional bodies including NICE Skills for Care and NHS England.[140,141,142] All health and social care professionals have to complete training and assessments in the safe administration and management of medicines and yet we still, as a society, get it wrong so often.

139 University of Manchester (2018) *More than 200 medication errors occur in NHS per year, say researchers* [online]. Available at: www.manchester.ac.uk/discover/news/more-than-200-million-medication-errors-occur-in-nhs-per-year-say-researchers/ (accessed August 2023

140 See www.nice.org.uk/guidance/sc1 and www.nice.org.uk/guidance/ng67 (accessed August 2023).

141 See www.skillsforcare.org.uk/Support-for-leaders-and-managers/Good-and-outstanding-care/inspection-toolkit/Topic-resources.aspx?kloe = safe-3&topic = medicine-optimisation&services = (accessed August 2023)

142 See www.england.nhs.uk/medicines-2/medicines-optimisation/ (accessed August 2023).

Evidence to support the Quality Statement

The regulation in this area requires far more than a policy and completed medicine administration records. It is worth noting that my book, *Towards Outstanding: Enabling Excellence in Care Home Provision*, provides resources for assessing and managing a service for continuous improvement that are relevant to any provider.[143]

Evidence from data and records

In terms of best practice, to make a service safer and ensure people are not harmed through poor practice rather than purely to appease a regulator, the documentary evidence needs to start, as ever, with an accessible current medicines management strategy and local policy, based on best practice guidance.

The policy needs to cover areas such as:

- Non-prescribed medicines and home remedies. Paracetamol for period pain in a learning disability supported-living environment, Clotrimazole anti-fungal cream for athlete's foot and simple cough linctus, where prescriptions are not necessary or even usual, but where the medication may make someone more comfortable.

- Self-administration of medicines where people have capacity to do so. People don't have to hand over all their everyday medicines when they are admitted to hospital, and care home residents may want to go out in the evening and take their diabetic medication with them.

- Covert administration of medicines is a necessary consideration for far more service types than just homes caring for people living with dementia. The prescribing doctor or other health care professional has responsibilities around prescribing for covert administration, and their own organisations' policies need to reflect this. Covert administration is a consent issue, and people usually have a right to make their own decisions about whether to take a drug or not. There are issues around capacity, best interest decisions and restraint. Each medicine must be considered separately, so a best interest decision to administer diuretics covertly, for example, does not allow for the covert administration of statins.

Apart from a policy, there are specific things that all providers will need to be able to evidence, including that staff who prescribe or manage medicines have access to the national guidance documents, such as the British National

---

143 See https://pavpub.com/health-and-social-care/towards-Outstanding-carehome (accessed August 2023).

Formulary and Midwives Exemption list. There may be a separate Midwives Exemption policy linked to the Medicines exemption policy. Under the Medicines for Human Use Act (2012), registered midwives may administer or supply, on their own initiative, any of the prescription-only medicines that are specified within Schedule 17, provided it is in the course of their professional midwifery practice.

There also needs to be evidence of a service-level agreement with a pharmacist, if the service does not directly employ their own pharmacists.

Medicines records and auditing

Providers need to ensure that there are records of the entire procurement, prescribing, storage, administration and disposal of medicines. That is where the involvement of a single GP practice and a single pharmacist service is of benefit to social care providers. Where care homes have more than one GP that they work with, and where they use several pharmacies, there is increased scope for errors. That does have the potential to limit the residents' choice, so should be discussed and the reasons explained when someone moves into a care home. If a resident still wants to see their 'own GP', consult with a private GP or use an online GP service, then they retain the right to do so. It is not for providers of adult social care to remove people's autonomy around medical care, but most people are happy to use the GP practice the provider contracts with.

Audit trail records are made easier by electronic monitoring, prescribing and supply systems that reduce the risks around inappropriate access and missed checks. Such systems vary in complexity and what they do, but the very best offer large providers the ability to see every time a drug storage area has been accessed and what was taken and by whom. They provide temperature monitoring and stock control facilities. They are usually outside the budget of most smaller providers, though.

If there is not a comprehensive electronic medicines control system, the provider needs to ensure that there are records for every step of the pathway, and that these are monitored to ensure the system is working effectively. That means delivery checks against orders, daily controlled drug stock checks with frequent management or pharmacist review of the controlled drug records, and an audit trail of controlled records such as HBP10 prescription pads and outpatient prescription pads. The monitoring of the HBP10 prescription pads needs a log of the numbers issued and to whom. The security checks can be completed by a manager walking around the premises at the end of the day and checking pads are all secured before leaving, or by an outpatient receptionist looking in each consulting room to check that none have been left lying around. The introduction of electronic prescribing and the printing of individual prescriptions has improved security, but there are still pads in use, and, where this is the case, there needs to be effective security.

Many providers have now moved to electronic prescribing with restricted access to the drug storage area and an electronic audit trail of access. This does make it much easier for managers and providers to be sure that medicines are being stored and accessed appropriately. It means illicit access and misuse can be identified much more quickly and acted on to prevent harm. It means there can be no debate about who took controlled drugs without signing the controlled drugs record. It makes stock control easier, and it reduces the risks of out-of-date medications being used. There are so many benefits that it becomes a worthwhile investment for larger providers, but again the cost is probably prohibitive for smaller services. Besides, the systems are good, but they are not the whole answer and staff can still make mistakes at every stage along the path. Providers need to understand the pathway and where errors are most likely to occur. Then they need to put in measures to minimise mistakes, react robustly when they do happen, and monitor the effectiveness of medication practices in the service.

Staff training

Every provider will be asked to provide training records around medicines optimisation at some point. There must be records showing that staff have received training appropriate to their role, whether that be experienced care assistants being trained in safe administration, registered nurses in adult social care being trained to support other staff and to complete audits or observations of practice, or an operating department assistant receiving training to enable them to ensure that best practice is followed in theatres. Those training records should include competency assessments when they are deemed necessary. Providers cannot rely on training in other services for this; even if a paramedic only works the odd shift and spends most of their time working for an NHS Trust, or an anaesthetist is only employed for one shift a week in a termination of pregnancy clinic, there need to be training records that show that staff have been trained around the provider's policies and practices.

There also needs to be a record of any additional training when something changes – whether that be the national guidance, the law, the prescribing system, or a new piece of equipment. Staff in a care home who have not used a syringe driver before may need to do so; the community nurses would usually provide that training (i.e. show them how) and that needs recording. An adult nurse working in a children's hospice may not have had to do many drug calculations previously, and so will need training and assessment to ensure that they are able to do the necessary maths processes.

Individual records also need to be completed accurately. Any gaps or changes must be clear, and all doses need signing for. Inevitably, there will be gaps, and these need to be investigated. That might be as simple as the nurse coming on duty at night seeing that the 6pm analgesia dose was not signed for and checking it was given. It needs recording as an incident in case it is happening often, and to understand whether it was simply that the resident was talking to a visitor at the time and the day nurse decided to wait then got caught up with something else, or whether staffing levels mean the day nurse was distracted and so busy they missed several people off the drug round.

Monitoring

The effectiveness of the policy needs monitoring, and there must be records of this. In a care home, that might be the registered manager or clinical lead checking all the individual medicines records each week for errors or omissions. It might be that the pharmacy contract includes monthly medicine optimisation audits by the pharmacist. Or it might be a diary entry showing that the electronic system was checked weekly to ensure that there was no access or removal of drugs that raised concerns.

Controlled drug books need monitoring to oversee the daily or shift checks, and that simply requires a signature and date in the book – by the matron, ward sister, clinical lead, pharmacist, registered manager or whoever else is meant to do it according to policy. While many checks and audits can be delegated to relatively junior staff, it may be better to ensure controlled checks remain with a more senior staff member who is in a position to act should anomalies be identified. Someone junior is possibly more likely to accept the word of a senior who dismisses their concerns and says it was just a counting error when there appear to be three vials unaccounted for. Using someone with professional registration to do these checks holds them professionally accountable, and so they are likely to ensure a more robust response to concerns.

An example – palliative care

A more recent example of medication error demonstrates the point that errors usually spring from systems issues rather than individual failings, and shows how systems not being used properly presented a risk to someone approaching the end of their life. The bulleted chronology below makes it easy to see how it could have been stopped and recorded as a 'near miss', showing that processes and safety measures were working:

- A busy specialist palliative care consultant mistakenly prescribes a dying patient 1,000 times the intended dose of an opiate to be delivered via a syringe pump.

- The ward nurse thinks this is a bit high, but since it was a consultant prescribing, she assumes it must be correct.

- The controlled drug cupboard does not contain enough of the drug. The nurse asks the ward sister who tells her to ring the pharmacy.

- The pharmacy says they don't have sufficient, so perhaps ask the adjacent hospice who will have plenty.

- The hospice matron says it is more than they usually give, but that particular consultant is very good and so it must be right.

- The hospice gives the ward nurse the controlled drugs after signing in the register.

- The nurse returns and gets a second nurse to witness the setting up of the syringe driver. The second nurse laughs about having to open so many vials and asks if the administering nurse is sure she has it right. The administering nurse replies that she has checked with the ward sister and the pharmacist.

- The witnessing nurse shrugs and signs the book. The administering nurse sets up the syringe driver.

- The consultant, meanwhile, is thinking about the patient and phones the ward to check they have calmed. The administering nurse says yes, they are now sleeping peacefully and laughs about needing to go to the hospice to get enough of the drug. The consultant digs a little and realises there has been a mistake somewhere. They return to the ward, check the chart and see their mistake in writing micrograms not milligrams. They stop the syringe driver shortly after it was set up and no harm is caused. It is duly reported and investigated. The finding is human error.

Was it a simple human error? How many opportunities were there to prevent the incorrect dose being administered? What systems changes could be made to ensure that the risk of repetition was reduced?

Evidence from staff and service users

Evidence from staff

Direct observation of staff practice is another very useful thing for managers and providers to do who want to deliver high-quality care. That is not about 'catching people out'; rather, it helps to understand where there are problems that impact on care delivery in relation to medicines management, and to spot any areas where practice could be improved. The findings should be discussed with individuals if there are specific concerns about their practice, but more useful would be to carry out a series of observations that allow usual practice and trends of poor practice. Knowing the areas where there are shortcomings means that efforts can be directed to making improvements that address those, rather than picking a random area to improve that may not actually make much difference.

As with most things, it is important to understand a problem before you try to solve it. If the observations show that a member of staff is being asked to carry out basic care while dispensing medicines to people, there may need to be staffing changes to ensure that there are enough staff to meet people's basic needs. If an operating department puts out unlabelled pre-filled syringes in a dish on a trolley before the list, there is scope for retraining and conversations about drawing up drugs at the time they are needed in team meetings. If staff are repeatedly interrupted while doing a medicine round, there may be a need for a reminder to other staff and the purchase of some 'Do not disturb' tabards. Understand what the problems are before trying to solve them.

The most recent case I have come across was a student nurse dispensing quite complex drugs unsupervised. The nurse in charge said the pots were checked to make sure they contained the right tablets before they were given to the patients. How a charge nurse can tell Oxycodone from Atenolol at a glance is hard to understand. How they would know which of their thirty-two patients were prescribed which drug is also hard to fathom. The truth is that they didn't, and they had become complacent. They risked their professional registration, the student's training and, most importantly, patient safety. It was almost certainly not a 'one-off' as the student was entirely unsupervised – it was usual practice, and regular observations of care would have shown that it was happening and provided an opportunity to address it.

If medicines management is high up the agenda and remains a key focus, then staff will tell the inspection team this. If they complete training around medicines management, they will say so – corroborating the documents the provider has available for inspection. If medicines errors are investigated, the individual and team receive feedback in some form and changes are made to reduce the risk of recurrence, this will reach the inspectors. While providers might encourage staff to say that everything is wonderful and they are a lovely team with a lovely manager and the home smells of roses, when asked direct, specific questions most people tell the truth. They might say all the lovely things – but then admit that sometimes people don't get their lunchtime medicines until nearly teatime because everyone is so busy, or there is only one registered nurse for eighty residents. Someone will inevitably say if people are told they aren't allowed to manage their own medicines, and it is quite likely that someone will proudly show one of the inspection team the very efficient system for putting all the intravenous drugs the anaesthetist wants drawn up in separate kidney dishes for each patient on a list.

Where there is safe care and treatment, staff will generally be very proud to talk about it. Providers just need to make sure their staff are proud of the quality of care and treatment they deliver, and feel able to raise concerns; it pays to talk to staff about specific areas of practice as well as the more general 'would you recommend working here to a friend?' Leaders should attend staff meetings and ask individuals how practice could be improved; then there will be no surprises when it comes to an inspection.

Evidence from service users

What about the views of the people using the service? Obviously, in many services, people aren't able to talk about the way their medicines are managed, but many are and do. They might mention, if asked, that the visiting GP ("that lovely Dr Elizabeth who comes in") goes through all their medicines and makes sure they are right. They might say they prefer the staff to sort all their medicines out, so they don't get in a muddle and make a mistake (which is a bit ironic given the level of medicines errors that occur). They might say they only need to ask for analgesia once and it appears. Conversely, if someone's mother is left with their Fentanyl patch unchanged for over a week and their daughter arrives to find them distressed and in pain, they will tell an inspection team or might even contact the Commission outside of an inspection. People misunderstand sometimes, and they might say they got pneumonia because of not having their cold treated properly, but on the whole they tell it as it is.

As with other areas of practice, speaking with people to ensure they understand and are happy with the way their medicines are managed is a good way to ensure that the policy is working. There are key questions that can be asked on a walk-around visit, when a triumvirate lead, regional director or senior manager speaks with service users, that help understand how well medicines are being managed to meet the needs of people using the service. It is that bit about 'meeting the needs of people using the service' that is key to this engagement-style monitoring. It's why medicines are prescribed and given – it's what actually matters, isn't it? What would you want in terms of medicines management if you were needing care or treatment? If there are discussions with people using the service, they should be recorded. Not their names or the details, but simply that "three people were asked whether their pain was well managed, and all said that it was. One person reported it being harder to get pain relief at night and that on their second post-operative night they had waited two hours for analgesia". That gives something to look at and work on to demonstrate that people are listened to and that what they say is used to improve the service.

Ultimately, having effective systems for care delivery, monitoring and improvement will result in better feedback – both from staff and from people using the service.

Part 4:
Conclusion

Chapter 19: Risk registers

Having thought about the risks that may present within a service, how they link to the regulations and Quality Statements, and what evidence could be used to show compliance, the final step is to ensure that there is some way of demonstrating those risks and that those risks are being monitored and addressed. It is entirely up to each provider how they do this, and it will vary depending on the size and scope of the service, but the usual expectation is that there will be a risk register.

There are tangible benefits to providers who use risk registers well to identify and address risk within their organisations. A risk register may act as an early warning signal, allowing providers to identify potential risks before they become serious issues. Spotting that one window restrictor is broken and rusty may prevent someone falling if the other restrictors are checked and replaced, if necessary. A risk register may also help with prioritising risks and determining the best course of action. Ignoring a dripping water pipe may prove very costly. Using a risk register in staff meetings or risk meetings improves communication between staff and those who are the decision-makers. It gives staff a voice and a route to raise concerns.

A risk register also gives ownership for actions and ensures that someone is responsible for monitoring and managing each risk. To quote a well-known story:

"Once upon a time, there were four people. Their names were Everybody, Somebody, Nobody and Anybody. Whenever there was an important job to be done, Everybody was sure that Somebody would do it. Anybody could have done it, but Nobody did it. When Nobody did it, Everybody got angry because it was Everybody's job. Everybody thought that Somebody would do it, but Nobody realised that Nobody would do it. So consequently, Everybody blamed Somebody when Nobody did what Anybody could have done in the first place."

Of course, the main reason for having a risk register is to develop ways of working that can reduce the likelihood and impact of potential risks and help to monitor risks over time. Since 2001, it has been mandatory for every NHS Trust in England to have a Board Assurance Framework. Most also have a corporate risk register – sometimes called an organisational risk register, Trust-wide risk register, or high-level risk register.

For adult social care services, the CQC says that for a 'Good' rating the provider will demonstrate that the service embeds a proactive approach to anticipating and managing risks to service users, which is recognised as being the responsibility of all staff. Staff understand the systems and strategies and use them consistently. Some aspects of the rating relate to individual risk, and they would not usually appear on a provider risk register, but the risks would be addressed in individual records. The 'Good' rating requires that the service focuses on improving its safety record, and that needs an effective risk-management process. Staff need to understand and use that process, which may be different for different risk types.

Monitoring and reviewing processes should enable providers and their staff to understand risks, and gives a clear, accurate and current picture of safety. It is the basis of good governance, and it is essential that, where increased risk is identified through monitoring the level of risk, the necessary actions to mitigate that risk are recorded. There is little point in having an action plan that is not monitored, or an identified risk that sits on a risk register for several years. Knowing that window restrictors are rusted and at risk of failing is of no use if nothing is done about it.

Types of risk register

What the risk register looks like is determined by the provider. For larger providers there will usually be several tiers of risk register, with operational units escalating the more serious risks upwards to a regional, department or divisional risk register where they are collated with other more serious risks from other operational units and the most serious of those risks are then escalated to the board, executive or provider. At each tier, those risks that are not escalated for higher level intervention or decision-making should not be ignored. They need to be addressed locally; staff need to know that local risk has been reduced or removed, and the actions need to be monitored to ensure that they are working. The same process happens at each level.

For some services, and particularly for NHS Trusts, the board and departmental risk registers are more complex and need to cover a range of risk types – including those related to patient care, workforce, finances, partnerships, estates, regulation, sustainability and IT infrastructure. Then there will be the 'add-on' risks around political and legislative or guidance changes – the impact of Brexit, COVID and changes of government priorities, for example. At present, there are risks around the changes to the national incident reporting and investigation processes as the new Patient Safety Incident Response Framework is rolled out, and risks related to the changes in regulation and a more responsive approach to risk from the Commission.

Sitting under the top-level risks seen by the board are a range of separate risks. To take an example, under patient care, the risks facing many acute hospital Trusts include long waiting lists leading to delayed diagnosis and treatment, insufficient capacity and high demand leading to handover delays from ambulances, people cared for in inappropriate settings, and poor or deteriorating outcomes. Some of those risks sitting under the headline risk will be managed at department or divisional level, while others need good oversight by the board. And this is where the Board Assurance Framework comes in, to identify any gaps in the assurance the board have around the risks that might prevent them delivering against their strategic objectives. By contrast, the corporate risk register comprises operational risks, mainly identified by services themselves. It does not include all the organisation's operational risks (a large NHS Trust will often have hundreds of these), just the most significant ones.

The risk management process

Whether the setting is a large and complex NHS Trust or a small care home with five residents, the process of managing risk is very similar and quite simple. The home may just have an Excel spreadsheet, whereas the Trust will likely have a system where local risks feed automatically into the next tier of risk register, but the fundamentals are the same. The starting point is a policy that covers risk management, and which is local to the service. It needs to be known and accessible to staff, and it should provide very clear guidance about how risks are managed and the levels at which decisions to address risk can be made, including those measures that involve additional costs.

Identify risks

Risks might be identified through monitoring compliance with policy, staff or people using the service reporting a concern, a complaint, staff or service user feedback, or from changes to national guidance, alerts or provider policies. Staff need to know how they can report and record risks – and understand that is what they are doing.

It might be there is a maintenance logbook where staff can write anything that needs mending – a soft tyre on a minibus, a fraying hoist sling or a cracked window. Alternatively, there might be a staff communication book where staff report that someone has phoned in sick, that a tray with used sharps was left on the side in the dirty utility, and that the visiting chaplain said that the lovely plant with shiny black berries in the garden looked like deadly nightshade but Mrs Livingstone thought they were nearly ripe blackcurrants.

These are risks that have been identified and staff need to recognise that language. A risk should always be described clearly in terms of its cause, what is likely to happen, and what impact it would have on the organisation if it occurred.

Assess the degree of risk

Some risks need immediate action – hopefully nobody would leave a smouldering mattress where someone had been smoking illicitly in their room while they went and read the policy and worked out the risk score.

Likewise, nobody would leave a shattered window on a children's ward until someone else read the maintenance log.

Other risks are less urgent, or there may be no quick fix. A GP practice with one receptionist off sick will need to ensure sufficient cover as a priority, but an NHS Trust with a 7.2% midwife vacancy rate will need to ensure adequate staffing to deliver safe care in the short term as well as addressing the risks associated with low staffing levels over the longer term.

Most provider risk registers have a scoring system that assesses risk in terms of impact and likelihood using the criteria set out in the organisation's risk management policy or process guidance. Risks should be prioritised, and those likely to cause immediate harm that can be addressed locally should be addressed locally. The local staff need to know how to do this and who has the authority to arrange for repairs, employ additional short-term staff, buy a takeaway if the oven breaks or buy additional fans in hot weather.

Address the risk – reduce or remove the risk

For every risk, controls should be listed – these are the measures that the organisation is already taking to reduce the level of risk. A risk register or risk management process should ideally have three scores recorded around each identified risk: firstly the inherent or underlying risk level score (the level of risk without any controls being introduced); secondly the current score (the level of risk remaining once the control measures are implemented); and thirdly the target score which the provider aims to reduce the risk to.

The controls need to be specific. If the mortality rate for a Trust is higher than expected and worsening, simply putting 'reduce mortality rate' is not addressing the risk. The actions should:

- Be specific, not vague.
- Address the risk.
- Be measurable.
- Have time limits or review dates.
- Have a named accountable person for each action.
- Have an overall lead where there are several actions required.

If an independent hospital offers a cancer care service which employs three chemotherapy-trained cancer nurse specialists and one goes on maternity leave, one is offered a promotion at the local NHS Trust and the other calls to say they are moving at the end of the month, there is a very clear risk that will likely score quite highly. There are risks around simply closing the service until staff can be recruited, as people may be in the middle of their treatment regimes, and there are risks associated with simply asking the surgical ward nurses to cover. In this example, local action may not be possible so the risk would probably be escalated to the regional risk register. That escalation needs recording, and staff need to know that it has happened. The regional team may be able to offer some benefit to staff at the closest hospitals to persuade them to provide cover in the short term until new staff can be recruited. They may also have the authority to employ suitably qualified agency nurses for three or six months.

Monitor and review the risk

Risk registers need to be working tools that reflect current unit, department, directorate, regional or organisational risk. Often, vague risks are identified and languish on risk registers for ever and a day. If there is a tiered risk-management process, the underpinning risk registers must be current in order that escalated risks are also current and to enable them to be addressed. Any risks that have diminished should be removed or have their score reduced.

Action taken at higher tier levels needs to be cascaded to operational staff to ensure they are aware how the risks in their area are being addressed further up the organisation – so, if a local team reports that there is a shortage of dairy produce in the weekly deliveries and this has been the case for three weeks, they might put a local action to go to a supermarket and use petty cash to top up the delivery. They would still escalate this risk if it continued, I imagine, and the provider risk register might show that the head of catering services for the group has arranged to meet with the supplier and review the contract. They might add they are exploring alternative providers. That risk would be reviewed in about a month and, if there are still problems, the catering manager might decide to arrange a specific contract with a local farm to provide all the dairy produce required. Another month of monitoring and the risk is reviewed again – the new farm supplier is working well, and staff report that their local cheese is very well received by service users. There is no longer a risk, so it is archived as no further action is necessary.

The inspection visit

When an inspection team visits, a risk register that is being used properly as a tool to record that risks are managed properly will serve as evidence that there are effective governance arrangements. In addition, staff will talk about their local risks and what is being done to reduce those risks, when asked. That's good for the rating but also good for staff. For example, if kept properly informed, they will know that, although there are staffing shortages, the provider is addressing these with a range of measures to improve recruitment and retention. They are more likely to speak positively when they know the provider is really trying to address the situation.

If middle managers or senior leaders are asked about the top three risks (i.e. those scoring highest on the risk register) in the organisation or their part of the organisation, they should know what they are because they are discussed and updates are shared. A director of nursing and midwifery who answers simply 'staffing, staffing, staffing', may indeed be very concerned about recruitment and retention, but they may not have good oversight of the increased incidents of infection or the risks to patient safety of frequently broken lifts to the operating theatres.

People using the service are unlikely to be asked about the risk register or the top organisational risks. They may be asked about how involved they are in planning their own care and what the management of their individual care is like. If broken lifts are on the risk register, they may be asked if they have used the lifts or had problems because of breakdowns, but generally this won't be discussed with service users.

Chapter 20: Summary

Managing risks is the key to safe care.

Health and social care is strewn with risks, from service-level risks such as failing premises and the use of high-risk substances such as controlled drugs, to the individual risks of complications of surgery, falls causing harm and the loss of freedoms. It is not possible to give a checklist that covers all types of risk in all provider types.

Each provider needs to think, as do its staff, as thinking practice is safer practice. There must be agreed ways of service delivery that follow national guidance and support best practice. Those ways of providing services are why there must be current policies that are reviewed and updated to reflect changes in the legislative or advisory requirements. Once policies have been agreed, they need to be shared, so that staff know what they say and work in accordance with them.

The ways in which care and treatment are delivered must be something all the staff understand and agree with if they are to 'buy in' to a commitment to excellence. Policies on a computer that staff cannot access are not much use; neither are policies that have been changed without those changes being shared. That means staff need training that enables them to understand what is required and why. Different roles and different grades of staff will need different training or different levels of training; a travel clinic receptionist will not need the same level of child safeguarding training as a consultant paediatrician.

Each provider needs to determine which staff need which training and that probably forms a policy on its own. Staff who understand the importance of people having clean spectacles and the risks of a greasy film blurring someone's vision are more likely to spend thirty seconds making sure they are clean when assisting people to dress each morning. Training records need to be maintained to allow the provider to retain oversight of who is trained and who isn't in any given area of practice. If training records are presented in a way that allows the data to be split by professional groups, by grades and by departments or sites, so much the better.

The provider needs to ensure that there are proper resources to enable the policy to be implemented and so reduce risks to people using the service. If there are no sharps boxes on the resuscitation trolley, staff will not be able to comply with the expected standard of used sharp disposal and the risk of needlestick injuries increases. If there are insufficient midwives on the delivery suite, they cannot be expected to maintain the supernumerary labour suite co-ordinator role and the one-to-one care required for women in established labour. If there are no thermometers to monitor bathwater temperature, then there is an increased risk of scalding. There needs to be a planned programme for equipment maintenance, for required checks, for replacement of items such as mattresses or pillows and for consumables, with a budget to allow the planned programme to be delivered.

Care and treatment delivery needs to be monitored to ensure that it is delivered in line with the provider's policies. That will vary depending on the policy and the service. It might mean documentary audits, observational audits, discussions in team meetings, monitoring of data over time to identify changing patterns in outcomes, or external reviews such as national audit programmes and checks such as MOTs and servicing of vehicles or independent pharmacy audits. When agreeing a policy, it is a good idea to include the monitoring arrangements that will be used to oversee the compliance and effectiveness of the policy. For some organisations, there will be external scrutiny and a requirement to submit data to other agencies, but that does not negate the need for each provider, and each leader of a given part of an organisation, to monitor the quality of care and treatment they or their team are delivering.

That means providers, managers and leaders checking how well they are complying with their own policies. Local Integrated Care Systems should have good oversight of all providers delivering NHS-funded care and treatment, but they are reliant on providers giving them information and data on their risks. If an independent hospital is not recognising that the framework around 'Never Events' applies to them, they will not report when a patient's face mask is connected to an air outlet instead of an oxygen outlet. If a care home manager is not reviewing (or checking a delegated person has reviewed) five recent incidents where visitors have reported that their relatives' fentanyl patches have 'fallen off', they might not see that the same member of staff was involved each time. The community pharmacist will not necessarily pick it up in a timely way to prevent further 'loss', and the local system leaders will only know if they are told. The inspection team, however, are very likely to pick it up.

Leaders and managers in organisations committed to learning and to safety will want to know that policies are followed, whether that be around checking that alternating air pressure-relieving mattresses are turned on, that the WHO Surgical Safety checklist is completed properly, or that people sitting out in the garden have sufficient shade. If problems are identified or policies are not being followed some or all of the time, action must be taken to improve the situation. If the policy isn't working, then there may be a need to review and amend it. If changes to practice mean that ambulance crews are required to divert to the least busy emergency department within a thirty minute drive, when the handover times at their default 'local' hospital are over four hours, on the say-so of the dispatch team, then the policy may need changing to reflect this. More often, the issue is around policy not being followed rather than an underlying problem with the policy itself.

In order to make improvements, providers need to understand why a policy is not followed. It is no use offering a labour ward coordinator two health care assistants and a phlebotomist if there are not enough midwives to provide one-to-one care in labour. There is little point in offering a vegetarian who complains of insufficient choice at lunchtime a cheese and ham toastie with the ham taken out (particularly if the cheese is not vegetarian). The first provider needs to understand why there is a shortfall against the planned numbers and address the underlying reason. The second needs to speak to the complainant to understand what choices have been offered, and then to the chef or catering manager to understand why there are such limitations.

Having understood the reasons why staff are not following policies, the provider (or its delegated representative) needs to develop an action plan that actually works and improves the situation. If there are repeated incidents involving a surgeon being very rude to staff in theatres and refusing to take part in the required WHO surgical safety checklist stages, all the posters in the staff room saying 'Be kind' are not going to do the trick. If this, along with a note about the importance of the WHO checklist in the monthly newsletter, is what is suggested (again) as a course of action, staff will simply feel they were not listened to. The action plan would be better addressing the problem directly, rather than tiptoeing around it. If three similar incidents or concerns have very similar action plans, then the action plan is probably not very effective.

Action plans need time constraints and responsible leaders for actions. They also need senior oversight and monitoring. If a Red, Amber, Green (RAG) rating system is used to show progress against the timeline and it is not mainly green, then there is a problem. Sometimes there is unavoidable slippage, but that should not be the norm. The norm should be providers, managers, leaders and staff who know the service, who recognise and address risks, and who are committed to delivering safe, personalised care to all.

To finish:

> "Let whoever is in charge keep this simple question in her head
> (not, how can I always do this right thing myself, but)
> how can I provide for this right thing to be always done?"
>
> Florence Nightingale[144]

---

144 Nightingale, F (1969) *Notes on nursing*. Dover Publications.

Appendix

Appendix

Regulation 12: 'Safe care and treatment'

This Appendix replicates in full the text of Regulation 12: 'Safe care and treatment'. The full text of other regulations and standards referred to in this book can be found on the website of the Care Quality Commission (www.cqc.org.uk).

Health and Social Care Act 2008 (Regulated Activities) Regulations 2014: Regulation 12

The intention of this regulation is to prevent people from receiving unsafe care and treatment and prevent avoidable harm or risk of harm. Providers must assess the risks to people's health and safety during any care or treatment and make sure that staff have the qualifications, competence, skills and experience to keep people safe.

Providers must make sure that the premises and any equipment used is safe and where applicable, available in sufficient quantities. Medicines must be supplied in sufficient quantities, managed safely and administered appropriately to make sure people are safe.

Providers must prevent and control the spread of infection. Where the responsibility for care and treatment is shared, care planning must be timely to maintain people's health, safety and welfare.

CQC understands that there may be inherent risks in carrying out care and treatment, and we will not consider it to be unsafe if providers can demonstrate that they have taken all reasonable steps to ensure the health and safety of people using their services and to manage risks that may arise during care and treatment.

CQC can prosecute for a breach of this regulation or a breach of part of the regulation if a failure to meet the regulation results in avoidable harm to a person using the service or if a person using the service is exposed to significant risk of harm. We do not have to serve a Warning Notice before prosecution. Additionally, CQC may also take other regulatory action. See the offences section for more detail.

CQC must refuse registration if providers cannot satisfy us that they can and will continue to comply with this regulation.

Note: The regulation does not apply to the person's accommodation if this is not provided as part of their care and treatment.

The regulation in full

12.—

1. Care and treatment must be provided in a safe way for service users.

2. Without limiting paragraph (1), the things which a registered person must do to comply with that paragraph include—

   a. assessing the risks to the health and safety of service users of receiving the care or treatment;

   b. doing all that is reasonably practicable to mitigate any such risks;

   c. ensuring that persons providing care or treatment to service users have the qualifications, competence, skills and experience to do so safely;

   d. ensuring that the premises used by the service provider are safe to use for their intended purpose and are used in a safe way;

   e. ensuring that the equipment used by the service provider for providing care or treatment to a service user is safe for such use and is used in a safe way;

   f. where equipment or medicines are supplied by the service provider, ensuring that there are sufficient quantities of these to ensure the safety of service users and to meet their needs;

   g. the proper and safe management of medicines;

   h. assessing the risk of, and preventing, detecting and controlling the spread of, infections, including those that are health care associated;

   i. where responsibility for the care and treatment of service users is shared with, or transferred to, other persons, working with such other persons, service users and other appropriate persons to ensure that timely care planning takes place to ensure the health, safety and welfare of the service users.

Guidance

This sets out the guidance providers must have regard to against the relevant component of the regulation.

12(1) Care and treatment must be provided in a safe way for service users.

Guidance on 12(1)

■ Providers must provide care and treatment in a safe way. In particular, this includes the areas listed in 12(2) (a) – (i). However, 12(2) is not exhaustive and providers must demonstrate that they have done everything reasonably practicable to provide safe care and treatment.

■ Providers should consult nationally recognised guidance about delivering safe care and treatment and implement this as appropriate.

12(2) without limiting paragraph (1), the things which a registered person must do to comply with that paragraph include–

12(2)(a) assessing the risks to the health and safety of service users of receiving the care or treatment;

Guidance on 12(2)(a)

■ Risk assessments relating to the health, safety and welfare of people using services must be completed and reviewed regularly by people with the qualifications, skills, competence and experience to do so. Risk assessments should include plans for managing risks.

■ Assessments, planning and delivery of care and treatment should:

▪ be based on risk assessments that balance the needs and safety of people using the service with their rights and preferences

▪ include arrangements to respond appropriately and in good time to people's changing needs

▪ be carried out in accordance with the Mental Capacity Act 2005. This includes best interest decision making; lawful restraint; and, where required, application for authorisation for deprivation of liberty through the Mental Capacity Act 2005 Deprivation of Liberty Safeguards or the Court of Protection.

All this applies when people use a service. This includes when they are admitted, discharged, transferred or move between services.

12(2)(b) doing all that is reasonably practicable to mitigate any such risks;

Guidance on 12(2)(b)

- Providers must do all that is reasonably practicable to mitigate risks. They should follow good practice guidance and must adopt control measures to make sure the risk is as low as is reasonably possible. They should review methods and measures and amended them to address changing practice.

- Providers should use risk assessments about the health, safety and welfare of people using their service to make required adjustments. These adjustments may be to premises, equipment, staff training, processes, and practices and can affect any aspect of care and treatment.

- Relevant health and safety concerns should be included in people's care and treatment plans/pathways. This includes allergies, contraindications and other limitations relating to the person's needs and abilities.

- Staff must follow plans and pathways.

- Medication reviews must be part of, and align with, people's care and treatment assessments, plans or pathways and should be completed and reviewed regularly when their medication changes.

- Providers must comply with relevant Patient Safety Alerts, recalls and rapid response reports issued from the Medicines and Healthcare products Regulatory Agency (MHRA) and through the Central Alerting System (CAS).

- Incidents that affect the health, safety and welfare of people using services must be reported internally and to relevant external authorities/bodies. They must be reviewed and thoroughly investigated by competent staff, and monitored to make sure that action is taken to remedy the situation, prevent further occurrences and make sure that improvements are made as a result. Staff who were involved in incidents should receive information about them and this should be shared with others to promote learning. Incidents include those that have potential for harm.

- Outcomes of investigations into incidents must be shared with the person concerned and, where relevant, their families, carers and advocates. This is in keeping with Regulation 20, Duty of candour.

- There must be policies and procedures in place for anyone to raise concerns about their own care and treatment or the care and treatment of people they care for or represent. The policies and procedures must be in line with current legislation and guidance, and staff must follow them.

- The provider must have arrangements to take appropriate action if there is a clinical or medical emergency.

- Medicines must be administered accurately, in accordance with any prescriber instructions and at suitable times to make sure that people who use the service are not placed at risk.

- When it is agreed to be in a person's best interests, the arrangements for giving medicines covertly must be in accordance with the Mental Capacity Act 2005.

- There must be arrangements to request a second opinion in relation to medicines for people who are detained under the Mental Health Act 1983.

12(2)(c) ensuring that persons providing care or treatment to service users have the qualifications, competence, skills and experience to do so safely;

Guidance on 12(2)(c)

- Staff must only work within the scope of their qualifications, competence, skills and experience and should be encouraged to seek help when they feel they are being asked to do something that they are not prepared or trained for.

- Staff should be appropriately supervised when they are learning new skills, but are not yet competent.

- Only relevant regulated professionals with the appropriate qualifications must plan and prescribe care and treatment, including medicines. Only relevant regulated professionals or suitably skilled and competent staff must deliver care and treatment.

12(2)(d) ensuring that the premises used by the service provider are safe to use for their intended purpose and are used in a safe way;

12(2)(e) ensuring that the equipment used by the service provider for providing care or treatment to a service user is safe for such use and used in a safe way;

Guidance on 12(2)(d) and 12(2)(e)

- Providers must ensure the safety of their premises and the equipment within it. They should have systems and processes that assure compliance with statutory requirements, national guidance and safety alerts.

- Providers retain legal responsibility under these regulations when they delegate responsibility through contracts or legal agreements to a third party, independent suppliers, professionals, supply chains or contractors. They must therefore make sure that these regulations are adhered to as responsibility for any shortfall rests with the provider.

- Providers should have and implement up to date induction and training plans for the safe operation of premises and equipment, including incident reporting and emergency and contingency planning.

- Providers should include in their financial planning the capital and revenue costs of maintaining safety.

- Providers must make sure that equipment is suitable for its purpose, properly maintained and used correctly and safely. This includes making sure that staff using the equipment have the training, competency and skills needed.

12(2)(f) where equipment or medicines are supplied by the service provider, ensuring that there are sufficient quantities of these to ensure the safety of service users and to meet their needs;

Guidance on 12(2)(f)

- People's medicines must be available in the necessary quantities at all times to prevent the risks associated with medicines that are not administered as prescribed. This includes when people manage their own medicines.

- Sufficient medication should be available in case of emergencies.

- Sufficient equipment and/or medical devices that are necessary to meet people's needs should be available at all times and devices should be kept in full working order. They should be available when needed and within a reasonable time without posing a risk.

- The equipment, medicines and/or medical devices that are necessary to meet people's needs should be available when they are transferred between services or providers.

12(2)(g) the proper and safe management of medicines;

Guidance on 12(2)(g)

- Staff responsible for the management and administration of medication must be suitably trained and competent and this should be kept under review.

- Staff must follow policies and procedures about managing medicines, including those related to infection control.

- These policies and procedures should be in line with current legislation and guidance and address:
  - supply and ordering
  - storage, dispensing and preparation
  - administration
  - disposal
  - recording.

12(2)(h) assessing the risk of, and preventing, detecting and controlling the spread of, infections, including those that are health care associated;

Guidance on 12(2)(h)

■ The Department of Health has issued a Code of Practice about the prevention and control of healthcare associated infections.[145] The law says that CQC must take the Code into account when making decisions about registration and by any court during legal proceedings about registration. By following the Code, providers will be able to show how they meet this regulation but they do not have to comply with the Code by law. A provider may be able to demonstrate that they meet this regulation in a different way (equivalent or better) from that described in the Code.

■ When assessing risk, providers should consider the link between infection prevention and control, antimicrobial stewardship, how medicines are managed and cleanliness.

12(2)(i) where responsibility for the care and treatment of service users is shared with, or transferred to, other persons, working with such other persons, service users and other appropriate persons to ensure that timely care planning takes place to ensure the health, safety and welfare of the service users.

Guidance on 12(2)(i)

■ The provider must actively work with others, both internally and externally, to make sure that care and treatment remains safe for people using services.

■ When care is shared between two or more providers or where there are integrated services, there should be appropriate arrangements to share relevant information promptly and in line with current legislation and guidance, and to plan and deliver care in partnership.

■ When more than one provider is responsible for the safety of a person using services, the responsibility for providing safe care rests with the principal care provider at the time it is given.

■ Arrangements should be in place to support people who are in a transition phase between services and/or other providers.

■ When people move between services or providers, appropriate risk assessments must be undertaken to make sure their safety is not compromised. This includes when they move between or with other bodies who may not be registered with CQC, such as the police. Decisions about a move between services or providers relating to people who may lack mental capacity to make that decision for themselves must be made in accordance with the Mental Capacity Act 2005.

■ To make sure that people who use services are safe and any risks to their care and treatment are minimised, providers must be able to respond to and manage major incidents and emergency situations. This includes having plans with other providers or bodies in case of events such as fires, floods, major road traffic accidents or major incidents, and natural disasters such as earth quakes or landslides (see the Civil Contingencies Act 2004).[146]

145 https://www.gov.uk/government/publications/the-health-and-social-care-act-2008-code-of-practice-on-the-prevention-and-control-of-infections-and-related-guidance
146 www.legislation.gov.uk/ukpga/2004/36/contents